Nutrition Made Clear

Roberta H. Anding, M.S.

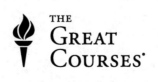

THE
GREAT
COURSES

PUBLISHED BY:

THE GREAT COURSES
Corporate Headquarters
4840 Westfields Boulevard, Suite 500
Chantilly, Virginia 20151-2299
Phone: 1-800-832-2412
Fax: 703-378-3819
www.thegreatcourses.com

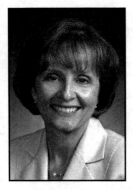

Roberta H. Anding, M.S., R.D./L.D., C.D.E., C.S.S.D.

Director of Sports Nutrition
and Clinical Dietitian,
Baylor College of Medicine
and Texas Children's Hospital

P rofessor Roberta H. Anding received her B.S. in Dietetics in 1977 and her M.S. in Nutrition in 1980 from Louisiana State University. She is currently a licensed dietitian in the state of Texas, a registered dietitian with the American Dietetic Association, a certified diabetes educator, and a certified specialist in sports dietetics.

Professor Anding began her career at the Tulane Medical Center and School of Medicine in 1982, where she was a part-time Assistant Professor and outpatient clinical dietitian education coordinator. She joined the faculty of the University of Texas School of Nursing at Houston in 1986 as Assistant Professor of Clinical Nursing. She later joined the faculty of Rice University as an instructor in the Department of Kinesiology, where she currently provides individual instruction to student athletes and teaches a course in nutrition. Professor Anding is an instructor in nutrition and is the clinical dietitian and director of sports nutrition in the Adolescent Medicine and Sports Medicine Clinic at Baylor College of Medicine. She is also currently the dietitian for the Houston Texans NFL franchise.

In graduate school, Professor Anding's research focused on the essentiality of omega-3 fatty acid in the development of the central nervous system. Her current research interests include the development of an online nutrition and fitness curriculum for inner-city Girl Scouts that was featured on the Houston Texans website. With grant funding from the Women's Fund, Professor Anding researched the development of a carbohydrate-modified weight management program for overweight Hispanic youth. She also received grant support from the Robinson Foundation for the innovative development of an educational DVD on weight management for adolescents.

Professor Anding has been honored with the Texas Dietetic Association's Texas Distinguished Dietitian Award in 2008 and its Media Award in 2006, the Houston Area Dietetic Association Media Award in 2004 and 2006, the Houston Area Dietetic Association Award for the Dietetic Internship Educator of the Year in 2001, and the John P. McGovern Outstanding Teacher of the Year Award while at the University of Houston School of Nursing. She has also been awarded the Houston Area Dietetic Association's Texas Distinguished Dietitian of the Year award several years running.

Throughout her career, Professor Anding has contributed to the publication of both scientific and consumer articles on nutrition and has authored several book chapters. She is a member of numerous state and local dietetic organizations, including the Sports and Cardiovascular and Wellness Nutrition Group of the American Dietetic Association. Professor Anding is the past chair of this national practice group. She is currently the American Dietetic Association media spokesperson for Houston, in which capacity she gives more than 100 media interviews per year. ■

Table of Contents

INTRODUCTION

Professor Biography i
Course Scope.. 1

LECTURE GUIDES

LECTURE 19
The DASH Diet—A Lifesaver... 3

LECTURE 20
Obesity—Public Health Enemy Number One.................................. 19

LECTURE 21
Healthy Weight Management 34

LECTURE 22
Metabolic Syndrome and Type 2 Diabetes................................... 51

LECTURE 23
Dietary Approaches to Weight Management................................... 67

LECTURE 24
Nutrition and Cancer Prevention 83

LECTURE 25
Nutrition and Digestive Health... 99

LECTURE 26
Prebiotics and Probiotics in Your Diet................................... 114

LECTURE 27
Food Safety—It's in Your Hands.. 127

LECTURE 28
Demystifying Food Labels 142

Table of Contents

LECTURE 29
Facts on Functional Foods 160

LECTURE 30
A Look at Herbal Therapy 175

LECTURE 31
Organic or Conventional—Your Choice 191

LECTURE 32
Fake or Real—Sugars and Fats 206

LECTURE 33
Creating Your Own Personal Nutrition Plan 223

LECTURE 34
Exercise and Nutrition—Partners for Life 242

LECTURE 35
The Future of Nutrition—Science and Trends 259

LECTURE 36
Nutrition Facts and FAQs 273

SUPPLEMENTAL MATERIAL

Glossary 290
Bibliography 304
Credible Nutrition Websites 324

Scope:

This course is an invitation to a journey to wellness—an inspirational, practical, hands-on guide to understanding the science of nutrition and how what we eat and drink affects our bodies and our lives.

We begin with a revealing study of why we eat what we do and how we gather information about nutrition. We then take an in-depth look at the core of our body—our digestive tract. We continue with a detailed review of the essential building blocks of diet and nutrition—protein, carbohydrates, fat, water, fiber, vitamins, and minerals—learning about their critical roles in a healthy diet.

The lectures then turn to topics critically important to the American public: the dietary links to major chronic diseases and disorders such as diabetes, hypertension, obesity, heart disease, and disorders of the digestive tract. The lectures are full of informative advice on what these illnesses are and practical suggestions for how we can lower our risk for acquiring them. The intent of the lectures is not to preach or scold but to present a wise but realistic approach to nutrition. Among the best—and most encouraging—advice in this course is "Progress, not perfection." In other words, even small changes toward improving our diet and exercise choices can make a big difference in our health.

In later lectures, we take a balanced look at the pros and cons of sugar substitutes and fat replacers, organic and conventional foods, and herbal therapies. We also cover topics from the importance of food safety to reading food labels (they are more complicated—and more important—than you think!). We survey the latest types of products on supermarket shelves (probiotics, prebiotics, and functional foods) and discover exciting new advancements in the science of nutrition.

In keeping with its goal to be relevant and beneficial for everyone, the course provides all we need to develop nutrition and exercise plans that not only work but are sustainable. After all, effective diet and nutrition choices cannot be quick fixes characterized by hunger and deprivation—they are lifestyle choices that can lead to a longer and healthier life for anyone at any age. ∎

The DASH Diet—A Lifesaver
Lecture 19

About 1 in 3 Americans faces hypertension, or high blood pressure. Uncorrected hypertension can lead to chronic renal failure, congestive heart failure, heart attack, stroke, and arterial aneurysm.

What constitutes high blood pressure? For adults, normal blood pressure is 120/80 millimeters of mercury. Systolic pressure is the top number, which is the force of the blood when the heart beats. Diastolic pressure is the bottom number, which is the force in between heart beats. Under the age of 50, the diastolic number is the focus; over 50, it is the systolic number. Prehypertension is defined as a blood pressure from 121/81 to 139/89 millimeters of mercury.

What are the risk factors for high blood pressure? Ethnicity is a risk factor. Up to 40% of African Americans have hypertension. Age is a risk factor. Physical inactivity can increase the risk of high blood pressure. People who are obese are at 5 times greater risk. Diets high in sodium and low in potassium or vitamin D increase risks. Sleep apnea is a common and often overlooked cause. Cushing's syndrome can cause high blood pressure.

Other atypical causes include nonsteroidal anti-inflammatory drugs. Other individuals at risk are pregnant women and individuals with polycystic kidney disease, kidney tumors, or insulin resistance. The stress of everyday life can also cause elevations in your blood pressure.

The DASH diet focuses on a high content of fruits, vegetables, and low-fat dairy products and a low fat composition.

What about the DASH diet? This total dietary approach to managing food is one example of the whole food approach that has been endorsed by the American Dietetic Association. With the addition of sodium restriction and weight management, there is strong evidence that this approach can and does work. In general, the DASH diet focuses on a high content of fruits, vegetables, and low-fat dairy products and a low fat composition.

What is the role of minerals and fats? For every 1-unit increase in the ratio of sodium to potassium excretion, there is a 24% increase in the risk of heart disease. Increasing calcium intake through supplements may actually increase the risk of heart disease and stroke in older women. Limiting saturated fat is great for the management of high blood pressure; increasing omega-6 and omega-3 fatty acids may also help control your blood pressure.

Here is an example of a DASH diet. Keep in mind these guidelines are based on calorie balance, but the general recommendation is that you should not consume less than the minimum number of servings in terms of portions.

- Eat 8 to 10 servings of fruits and vegetables a day to drive up potassium intake. Eat 6 to 8 servings of whole grains.

- Consume 2 to 3 servings of dairy—generally skim or low-fat milk or yogurt. Consume about 6 ounces of lean protein, including chicken and fish.

- Have about 2 to 3 servings of oil or other fats, including olive oil, peanut oil, safflower oil, and sunflower oil.

- Aim for 4 to 5 servings of beans, nuts, or seeds per week.

Let's review some frequently asked questions. My food does not taste salty; does that mean I have a low-sodium diet? No, just because a food does not taste salty does not mean it is low in sodium.

If I have to eat 8 to 10 servings of fruit, can I just drink more juice? By drinking more juice, you do get more potassium in your diet, but keep in mind the bigger picture—eating the whole fruit will give you more fiber and better control over portion size.

Is the DASH diet something that my whole family can do? Your whole family can be on this diet.

Is there anything that I can do to make food preparation easier? Make meals using whole ingredients, and when you do need to buy fast food, look for fruit or vegetable options.

Are there cookbooks for this diet? Anything from the American Heart Association integrates all this science and puts it into a usable form for consumers. The National Heart, Lung, and Blood Institute also has DASH recipes. For more examples of the DASH diet, go to http://www.dashdiet.org/. ∎

Suggested Reading

McArdle, Katch, and Katch, *Exercise Physiology*, chap. 2.

Questions to Consider

1. What aspects of the DASH diet do you already incorporate in your life?

2. What aspects of the DASH diet would you find most challenging to incorporate in your life?

The DASH Diet—A Lifesaver
Lecture 19—Transcript

Welcome. I'll start off by telling you a story. I had an elderly woman who came into my clinic, who had high blood pressure and she was really fearful of making a wrong food mistake. So she was limiting her portion sizes. She had cut out salt. But she came in and shared with me a great strategy she had. She was modifying her favorite meatloaf recipe. She'd given up the salt in the meatloaf, but actually, what she was putting in was Worchester sauce, ketchup, barbeque sauce, all of those are really high-sodium foods. We talked about modifying her meatloaf and talked about the hidden sources of sodium in that meatloaf. We modified it. We increased her portion sizes and quite honestly, we had a better outcome. She was eating a little bit more, which she needed to do, and she ended up having an improvement in her nutritional status.

Hypertension or high blood pressure is one of the most pervasive, chronic disorders facing Americans. According to the National Center for Health Statistics and the National Heart, Lung, and Blood Institute, the prevalence of hypertension in the United States varies by ethnic group. It's an unbelievably prevalent disorder with millions of Americans being affected, and over 1 billion people worldwide every year are diagnosed with high blood pressure. Here in the United States, that equates to one-out-of-three Americans, really a very pervasive disorder.

What are the consequences? Uncorrected high blood pressure can lead to congestive heart failure, heart attack, stroke, arterial aneurism, where the walls of the blood vessel become dilated, and it is the leading cause of chronic kidney or renal failure in the United States, leading to dialysis. Even a moderately elevated blood pressure can lead to a shorter life expectancy. I'm going to remind you not everybody has signs and symptoms of high blood pressure, so you really have to monitor. There is a solution out there, and the solution is called the "DASH diet." "DASH" stands for "Dietary Approaches to Stop Hypertension."

There are many dietary strategies to control high blood pressure, and that's good news for all of us because now we're armed with lots and lots of tools. We've got weight management, adequate potassium, calcium, and magnesium are central to managing your blood pressure. Now, remember, those are the nutrients that we're going to concentrate on, but we're also going to integrate that with food.

What constitutes high blood pressure? For adults, normal blood pressure is considered 120 over 80 millimeters of mercury, and that's your normal blood pressure. What is blood pressure? Blood pressure is the force of the blood pumping against the arterial walls. Sometimes this is defined as cardiac output, how hard the heart is pumping, and peripheral resistance, what kind of resistance does that blood meet as it flows through the blood vessels. Even slight elevations above this number can cause health problems.

That systolic number is the top number, and previously, it was thought this is not a very important number. We don't really know the magnitude or the effect of high systolic pressure, but that's the force of the blood when the heart beats. Most recently, multiple studies suggest that decreasing that systolic blood pressure by 12 to 13 millimeters of mercury over a four-year period of time can reduce the incidence of stroke by 37%. The take-home message is that top number matters. It matters and it matters in a big way.

Diastolic pressure is the bottom number. It represents the force in between heart beats. It's a more important risk factor for those under the age of 50. According to the American Heart Association, the pattern and significance of high blood pressure changes depending on your age. So under the age of 50, you may focus on the diastolic number. Over the age of 50, it's the systolic number. Both of these numbers are important.

The systolic number often represents the stiffness of those blood vessels. So again, as we age, as we end up with plaque in our arteries, all of those risk factors stiffen that blood vessel slightly and again, increase that systolic number. For those individuals who have normal blood pressure at 55—if you are 55 or older and you said, "I have normal blood pressure, I don't have a risk factor"—I'm going to encourage you to continue to monitor because you still have a 90% lifetime risk of high blood pressure. You might be lulled into this false sense of security—"I'm good to go because my systolic number is great and I'm 57 years old"—monitor, monitor, and monitor. This stress on monitoring is according to the Seventh Report of the Joint National Committee on the Prevention, Detection, Evaluation, and Treatment of High Blood Pressure. Their suggestions are that for every 20 millimeter mercury rise in systolic pressure and 10 millimeter mercury rise in diastolic pressure, you double the risk of heart disease. That's why this monitoring makes a difference.

We now have a new category that's not really a disease, but it's, again, that early warning sign that your body's giving you, that flashing light on the dashboard that says pay attention. Pre-hypertension is defined as a blood pressure from 121 over 81 to 139 over 89 millimeters of mercury. Not a disease category, but it tells you who's at risk of developing hypertension. I'm going to suggest to you, follow the science on this because as the science emerges, this category may become more relevant over time.

What are the risk factors? The risk factors for high blood pressure are numerous. Ethnicity is one. Depending on the estimates that you read, up to 40% of African Americans have hypertension. They oftentimes develop, as an ethnic group, hypertension earlier, and it's a more severe and often more difficult form to treat. We don't really have a good reason why African Americans are more vulnerable. Again, if you are African American, please make a note that not only do you need to check your blood pressure, but your children's blood pressure, regardless of their weight, regardless of other risk factors.

We know about age. According to the National Heart, Lung, and Blood Institute, again, over the age of 55, normal blood pressure, you can still have an increased lifetime risk. Hypertension or high blood pressure itself is defined as when your blood pressure is consistently higher than 140 over 90. Now, we've all had experiences when we're anxious or nervous, you're going to that new doctor for the first time, and they say, "oh, your pressure is high." Remember that isolated one blood pressure is not what we're looking at. We're looking at a pattern over time.

Physical inactivity can increase the risk of high blood pressure. How much exercise do you need to have? A major study looking at 54 individual studies on the dosing of aerobic exercise demonstrated that at all levels and all intensities, regular aerobic exercise can lower that top number, the systolic number, by 3.8 millimeters of mercury, and the diastolic by 2.6. Keep in mind, however, if the exercise goes away, so will the beneficial effects. We've all heard the adage "an apple a day keeps the doctor away." I'm going to suggest we have a new one, "a walk a day keeps the pressure away."

Diet and nutrition as risk factors. People who are obese are at five times greater risk of developing high blood pressure. According to one study, obese women are more likely to have an increase in systolic pressure than men. So it appears that there may be some gender discrimination there. Central obesity is a key finding. Are we seeing a trend here yet? The trend is that obesity is going to contribute to most of our chronic diseases, but in this case, I'm going to encourage you to get out your tape measure so we can get this up close and personal.

Here's what you do. Take your tape measure and measure around the level of your belly button. If you are a male and your waist circumference is greater than 40 inches, you're going to have an increased risk of high blood pressure. For women, if your waist circumference is greater than 35 inches, you have an increased risk. So it's not only are you overweight, it's where is your weight clustered? Sometimes you'll see this as the difference between an apple-body shape, abdominal obesity, and a pear-body shape, where you have your weight in your hips and thighs. We know that overweight or obesity is going to be a risk factor in terms of diet and nutrition.

People who consume diets high in sodium and low in potassium are more likely to develop hypertension. Now here again, what we're seeing is a trend that we have in this case two minerals that act in opposition to one another. We've seen that with insulin and glucagon in terms of hormone, and this is going to come up over and over again in clinical nutrition. That diet high in sodium versus a diet low in sodium is also going to contribute to high blood pressure.

Vitamin D may play a role. Individuals with vitamin D deficiency are found to have a higher than average systolic and diastolic blood pressure. Who would have thought even five years ago that having adequate amounts of vitamin D may also reduce your risk of having high blood pressure?

Certainly, individuals who have a family history of high blood pressure are more likely to develop high blood pressure. So a lot of the chronic illnesses that we're exploring have not only a dietary and environmental cause, but have a genetic cause as well.

Sleep apnea, however, is a common and oftentimes overlooked cause of high blood pressure. Sleep apnea occurs when you can't get adequate oxygen delivery and you are waking up multiple times during the night. Now, you might not actually be aroused from sleep, but the key finding here is ask your partner whether or not you snore. If you snore, you're much more likely to have sleep apnea. Of course, I would never snore, so my husband would say, "absolutely not."

Cushing's syndrome, an unusual cause of high blood pressure, occurs when you have an over-secretion of the hormone cortisol, and that can cause high blood pressure. Other atypical causes include certain popular drugs, such as non-steroidal anti-inflammatory drugs such as aspirin or ibuprofen, can cause high blood pressure, but keep in mind that's not a typical cause.

Other individuals are at risk of developing hypertension and those are individuals who are pregnant, individuals with polycystic kidney disease, kidney tumors, insulin-resistance, and again, this is a recurring theme. Too much insulin, remember insulin is an anabolic hormone, in this case helps us to retain or hang onto that additional sodium. Certainly, we all know the stress of everyday life can also cause elevations in your blood pressure, so a holistic view might be that you not only need to walk, and you need to monitor your diet, but you also need to integrate strategies to reduce stress in your life.

What about the DASH diet? Do we have any solutions here? Again, many dietary strategies can be implemented to control high blood pressure, and oftentimes the combination of one or more strategies can lead to a better result. This total dietary approach of managing food, not necessarily supplements, is one of the best methods to communicate a health and nutrition message. The DASH diet is one example of the whole food approach that's been endorsed by the American Dietetic Association.

The question is does it work? The original DASH diet did not stress sodium restriction or even body fat management, and the results were equivocal. Some studies would say, yes, the DASH diet works, and others said no. With the addition of sodium restriction and weight management, there is strong evidence that this approach can and does work. Research using the DASH diet to treat hypertension shows it can lower blood pressure in some people, not those that have very resistant high blood pressure, oftentimes not as effective in African Americans. It can lower blood pressure to the same extent as drug therapy does. It can also lower blood pressure often more than other lifestyle changes, and again, more than one singular intervention alone.

The bottom line here is combining all these strategies and not just picking one, not just focusing on sodium restriction, is more effective than a combination of other lifestyle strategies. After two months on this diet, when individuals are put on the DASH diet, what have we seen? We've seen a reduction of systolic pressure by an average of 11.4 millimeters of mercury, and a diastolic decrease by 5.5 millimeters of mercury. Very significant. For every 2 millimeters of mercury reduction in systolic pressure, it reduces your risk of heart disease by 5% and your risk of stroke by 8%. I'm not a gambling woman, but I tell you, I will take those odds any day, that if I can introduce a dietary approach that's going to be helpful, I'm really going to get on board with that.

Other results of lowering your blood pressure can include reducing the risk of progression of dementia and other cognitive impairments. These disorders are more common in those individuals who have high blood pressure. Now, again, this moderation of alcohol comes up just like it has come up in the prevention of cardiovascular disease, but any more than moderate amounts of alcohol can actually have the reverse effect. It can increase pressure. Again, we've got to define moderate. Moderate means one glass of wine for women, two glasses of wine for men. But portions always rule. A portion is about a five-ounce glass for wine. You have to think of what is the size of your wineglass at home? If you're not sure, measure it, and if your standard wineglass is eight ounces, that's more than one glass of wine, according to the science on standardized portions.

Further research has shown that the standard DASH diet combined with dietary sodium or salt restriction is going to be even more effective. Now, I'm going to tell you the science will suggest if you combine that with 1500 milligrams of sodium or less, you can get really even more significant reductions. I have to tell you though that's a bit of a difficult challenge for most Americans, as we're going to explore. Again, adding in some sodium restriction can be helpful, but just like my elderly woman, if it gets to the point where you cannot tolerate the way your food tastes, adding a little bit more salt may actually improve your nutritional status because we've got lots of tools in our toolbox in terms of controlling high blood pressure.

In general, the DASH diet focuses on a high content of fruits, vegetables, low-fat dairy products, and a low-fat composition. I'm going to suggest to you, however, we're not just talking about low fat. We're talking about right fat, and remember those right fats tend to be the essential fatty acids, omega-6 and omega-3 fatty acids.

What's the role of potassium, the major mineral in fruits and vegetables? Sodium and potassium are the yin and yang of blood pressure nutrition. Again, I'm going to suggest that you listen to the lecture on those minerals. For every one-unit increase in the ratio of sodium/potassium excretion, how much you're getting rid of, there was a 24% increase in the risk of heart disease. Lowering the sodium intake while increasing the potassium intake is the best stroke defense. The analogy I use is bodies like to be in the middle of the road. We really like the middle of the road. It gives us a little wiggle room. We can go left or right a little bit, but when I have a high sodium intake and a low potassium intake, I've got an imbalance here. My body is forced to live in the ditch, and we don't do very well as humans when we live in the ditch. We're designed to go down the middle of the road.

Keep in mind what we're trying to do is really balance those minerals. The hard part is the average American consumes about 3.6 grams of sodium per day. This is more than the federal guidelines of 2.4 grams of sodium per day. The American Heart Association gets a bit more aggressive and recommends under 2 grams of sodium per day. However, sodium and salt are not really the same thing, but we use those things interchangeably. Salt, by definition, is sodium times 2.5, and many of us use these terms interchangeably. A teaspoon of salt is equal to 2.3 grams of sodium, so again, just a teaspoon of salt in your diet a day is going to be close or exceed most of our public health recommendations on sodium consumption.

The other challenge is that most Americans consume less than the 4.7 grams of potassium that's recommended per day. There are lots of estimates out there. Current estimates are that Americans only consume about 3 grams per day. So again, we've got this imbalance of sodium and potassium, and what we're trying to do is bump those up. Here's a key point for you. Diet should include less processed food to decrease the sodium because keep in mind when we're talking about high blood pressure, we're really talking about the sodium and not just the salt. So the more processed a food is, in general, the more instant a food is, the higher the sodium content. Again, that food may not taste salty, but there's sodium built in.

Diet should increase the amount of fruits and vegetables. Here's another great question. How can I make my food taste good without salt? The challenge is as we age, our sense of taste evolves and some people would say it actually diminishes. In essence, to taste the food, we need more sodium to flavor and taste our food. Again, my elderly woman who was trying to reduce the sodium content of her meatloaf didn't like it without the salt, and part of that was because of her age. However, most of us believe less salt equals less delicious. There are some things that you can do to improve the flavor. Certainly, you can use lots of different spices and herbs, and one of my favorite is using hot sauce. You can use Tabasco and hot sauce. Yes, there's sodium in that hot sauce, but practically speaking, you can't use enough of that for that to be a significant sodium load.

Foods can be spicy if you like spicy food. They just can't be salty. Again, one of my favorite things to do is take liquid crab boil, and when I'm boiling potatoes, I put a little crab boil in the potatoes, and it gives it this wonderful seasoned flavor, but is not salty.

What about other minerals, besides sodium and potassium? Does that make a difference? Some recent studies suggest that increasing calcium intake may actually increase the risk of heart disease and stroke in older women. Wait a minute here. Isn't the DASH diet focusing on low-fat dairy products?

The answer is yes. Aren't dairy products a great source of calcium? Yes. However, I'm going to suggest that this study was in the case with those who had emerging kidney failure and it's almost always in individuals who are taking calcium supplements, not calcium from food. It's really difficult to get too much calcium from food. So again, when the American Dietetic Association stresses a whole food approach and not a supplement approach, here's the reason why. Because with a supplement, I can very easily get my calcium intake above what is practically going to be consumed in diet. Again, the bottom line here is that too much or too little with calcium can affect blood pressure. I would encourage you not to consume an excessive amount of calcium from supplements, which will be defined later.

We know that limiting saturated fat is also a great idea in the management of high blood pressure. Why is that the case? Keep in mind saturated fat helps you to deposit plaque in arterial walls because it triggers the synthesis of cholesterol. If high blood pressure is cardiac output times peripheral resistance, the combination of those two, the more plaque in my arteries, the more resistant to that blood flow my body becomes. Increasing omega-6 and omega-3 fatty acids may also help to control your blood pressure. Remember, both of these are essential. In our American diet, we tend to eat too much omega-6 and not enough omega-3, but remember our bodies crave balance.

Can we give you an example of a DASH diet? Yes, there's a wonderful example of how you can implement this in your guidebook. Again, I'm going to suggest to you that the DASH diet is based on calorie levels and quite honestly, you really need to match your calories because the portion sizes that are recommended on the DASH diet are almost always going to be linked with energy balance. Again, if you're more physically active, you should boost your portion sizes or the number of items to maintain your weight. If you're looking to lose weight, you might have to adjust your calories. Keep in mind these guidelines are going to be based on calorie balance, but the general recommendation is that you should not consume less than the minimum number of servings that I'm going to give you in terms of portions for the DASH diet.

Again, depending on your calorie needs, it's going to vary, but the key point is a significant increase in fruits and vegetables. This is how we're going to drive that potassium intake up. In general, again, depending on calorie balance, we're looking at 8 to 10 servings of fruits and vegetables a day, and you're going to think, "oh my, there's no way I can do that." Keep in mind that a serving is half a cup, and if you're trying to estimate, a half a cup is about the size of the palm of your hand. If you have a big bowl of grapes, that could honestly be two servings right there. Six to eight servings of grains, and I'm going to ask you the question, "what kind of grains are we talking about?" Of course, the answer is whole grains. Two to three servings of dairy. Again, what is a serving? It is an eight-ounce glass. If you're not sure how many ounces you have in a standard glass in your own home, measure it. The dairy servings are generally fluid milk, skim or low fat, or skim or low-fat yogurt. Technically speaking, cheese is considered a dairy portion, but because of the high saturated fat content, it really is going to get bumped to the side on the DASH diet.

Somewhere in the range of six ounces of lean protein, and that's going to be chicken, fish. Remember, any meat that has the word "loin" in the name is going to be considered a lean protein. Three ounces of meat, again, is about the size of the palm of your hand, or the size of a deck of cards. You could very easily get six ounces of lean protein in a meal. Again, when we talk about servings, they are standard servings. It's not necessarily what you're serving yourself on your plate. Somewhere in the range of two to three servings of oil or other fats, but please always remember what we're looking for are mono- or polyunsaturated fats, so olive oil, peanut oil, safflower oil, sunflower oil would all be good examples of how to add fat to your diet. Also aim for four to five servings of beans, nuts, or seeds per week, not per day.

I think the challenge here is, can we integrate this? The answer is yes. If you think about the DASH diet, with the exception of the addition of the sodium restriction and really trying to amp up the fruits and vegetables, this really fits most public health guidelines. We're tweaking this to take the science of what we know about these individual minerals, and what we're now trying to do is combine that into an eating plan that you can enjoy.

Frequently asked questions. My food doesn't taste salty, so that means I have a low-sodium diet? I can't taste the salt in my food. That's the hard part because the answer to that is no. Keep in mind "instant" or "processed" generally means higher levels of sodium. My favorite example is two or three years ago, there was a brand of pudding on the market that you could just add water to and shake it. Now, remember you can make pudding by using skim or low-fat dairy products. You can make it homemade. You can make the pudding that takes 24 hours to set, or you can make this instant pudding. The sodium content from the homemade pudding is about 120 milligrams of sodium, to the middle of the road at about 300 milligrams of sodium, to the instant pudding at 590 milligrams of sodium. So it's a great example as I go from less processed to more processed, what's going to happen? The sodium content of my diet is going to rise.

Just because a food tastes salty doesn't mean it's a high-sodium food. The salt could be on the outside. This one may surprise you. A small vending machine size bag, not a grab bag, not a bigger bag, but a small individual bag of potato chips, has in the range of about 150 milligrams of sodium, so it's actually significantly less than that instant pudding. It tastes salty because the sodium is on the outside. That is the reason it tastes salty. Again, sometimes you can be a little bit misled. Go back to that nutrition facts panel and look at the sodium that's added because remember, the sodium can be sodium chloride, table salt. It can be sodium propionate as a food additive. It can be baking soda, sodium bicarbonate. There can be lots of places where there's sodium sneaked in and the food doesn't necessarily taste salty. Again, it's the sodium content that rules. We think sodium and salt are interchangeable terms. They are not, and so you want to look at the label for sodium intake.

If I have to eat 8 to 10 servings of fruit, can't I just drink more juice? Keep in mind what we're really trying to do here is an integrated approach, and yes, by drinking more juice I can get more potassium in my diet, and that may be a strategy for some people that just can't tolerate the volume. What we're really looking for is this integrated approach. If I need to lose weight, if losing weight is going to be an effective intervention to control my blood pressure, I don't necessarily want to over-drink juice and not pay attention to portion size. Portion size rules. Portion sizes are king. I think that's a really key strategy. Yes, you can drink more juice, but in my world, I'd much rather have you eat the whole fruit. Again, I'm getting fiber and I'm going to get other things that are going to make that diet a little bit more integrated and holistic.

Is the DASH diet something that my whole family can do, or is there anything that I can do to make the food preparation easier? The answer is yes, your whole family can be on this diet. Keep in mind you want things that are less instant, so for example, most days of the week, you can make a meal for your family and you're using whole ingredients. A couple of days a week, you really need to go out and get fast food. You think, okay, I'm going to go out and get fast food. I'm going to go out and get a burger. Well, I kind of know that's probably going to be relatively high in sodium, but maybe in this fast food restaurant, I'll look for a fruit or vegetable option. This could be a great time to see whether or not they're selling orange juice on their menu. Can you get sliced apple? Think fruits and vegetables to kind of balance out that high sodium.

Keep in mind that your body remembers what you do most of the time. Just like in the management of high blood pressure, it's not that singular value that we're concerned about. We're looking at changes over time, and your body works the same way. If you have to have a higher sodium meal because of your family demands, so be it. Keep in mind, because this is a whole food approach, and certainly, most Americans are going to develop high blood pressure in their lifetime, why not put your three- or four-year-old daughter, son, grandson, granddaughter on this diet? It's perfectly fine for them. It is a wellness approach for your whole family. Most of the time, we consume more sodium than we need, and so teaching our children that fruits and vegetables and grains can be delicious without salt is a gift that only you can give them.

Are there cookbooks out there? Are there any cookbooks that are out there? I'm asked that question all the time. I'm going to suggest to you anything from the American Heart Association, whether it's online, or whether it's an American Heart Association cookbook, really integrates all this science and puts it into a usable form for consumers. Another great place to get great information is the National Heart, Lung, and Blood Institute, and they actually have DASH pamphlets, DASH recipes, and some other ways that you can quickly get on board with this DASH approach.

Monitoring your high blood pressure, and realizing that you can be an integral part in controlling your high blood pressure, takes you on that road to wellness. Thank you.

Obesity—Public Health Enemy Number One
Lecture 20

Often cited as public health enemy number one, obesity has been on a steady rise since the early 1970s. Children and adolescents are the age group getting the biggest the fastest.

We are going to tackle the subject of overweight and obesity. The challenge with this topic is how to get ourselves more centered in our approach to overweight and obesity. Let's start with a few definitions. Overweight is defined as a body mass index (BMI) between 25 and 29.9. Obesity is a BMI of 30 or greater. Overfat refers to people who have a normal BMI but are carrying more of their weight as body fat.

Obesity is now a global problem. It contributes to ill health as the top global nutrition-related problem and is on the rise in every country in the world. A study in *The New England Journal of Medicine* suggests that any dietary strategy can work, but you have to stick with it. Children and adolescents are concerned with weight but do not recognize diet and calorie management as effective strategies.

[Obesity] contributes to ill health as the top global nutrition-related problem and is on the rise in every country in the world.

Let's look at factors in the development of obesity. There are biological factors: When both parents are morbidly obese, there is an 80% chance their children will be obese. It is estimated that your genetic makeup can account for 50%–90% of the variations in your ability to store body fat. Fat cells play a role in the development of obesity: hypercellular obesity, hypertrophic obesity, and hyperplastic obesity. Sex, age, and ethnicity all play a role in weight gain. There is also a science of satiety, which is under the control of 2 relatively newly discovered hormones, leptin and ghrelin.

Social and environmental factors can play a role in the development of obesity. Americans are more likely to be obese if they have a low socioeconomic status. Level of education is associated with body weight as well, but mostly only for women. The media also plays a role. Another factor is our built environment—for instance, whether our neighborhoods are walkable. Social factors also affect the way that we choose our food. There are lifestyle and behavior factors as well: Lack of exercise is a major factor contributing to obesity. There are also psychological factors: People eat to cope with stress or alleviate boredom.

How do we know if we are overweight? BMI is the gold standard of population-based measurements of overweight. A BMI of less than 24.9 is considered normal weight, between 25 and 29.9 is overweight; 30 or greater is obese. BMI is not necessarily the best tool for evaluating all individuals.

What about the health risks of being overweight or obese? The longer the obesity persists, the higher the risks. Overweight people are 2 to 6 times more likely to develop hypertension. Overweight people have increased risk for stroke, deep vein thrombosis, impaired cardiac function, high blood triglycerides, low HDL, insulin resistance, and type 2 diabetes. Obesity can be a risk factor for the development of cancer. Obese people are more likely to have degenerative joint disease; sleep apnea and mechanical breathing constraints, particularly during exercise; problems with anesthesia during surgery; and compromised wound healing. Other risks include gallbladder disease and nonalcoholic steatohepatitis. There is also a psychological burden: depression, stigmatization, bullying, and discrimination.

Losing weight can reduce disease biomarkers. People who are obese and lose as little as 5%–10% of their body weight can improve their blood pressure, insulin levels, glucose, cholesterol, and triglycerides. Health-care professionals treat obesity like a disease and will emphasize health and fitness over what you should weigh.

Let's review some frequently asked questions. What is weight cycling? Weight cycling is a pattern of losing and regaining weight repeatedly. There is an antidiet movement advocating for size acceptance. What do you think about that? I think psychologically it is a good thing, but with size acceptance, often we are not calling obesity what it is—a disease. ∎

Suggested Reading

McArdle, Katch, and Katch, *Exercise Physiology*, chap. 30.

Questions to Consider

1. Why is obesity called public health enemy number one?

2. Why do you believe the incidence of obesity has increased so dramatically in the United States in recent years?

Obesity—Public Health Enemy Number One
Lecture 20—Transcript

Welcome back. In this lecture, we're going to tackle the weighty subject of overweight and obesity. I'm going to start out by giving you kind of an update of the state of affairs.

At Texas Children's, we have started a bariatric surgery program for adolescents, given the rising girth of our nation. We had a young lady who was coming in and she had a BMI, which we'll talk about in a little bit, a BMI of close to 50. The question that we toyed with is, how are we going to teach her about her diet? We talked about her pre-op diet and her post-op diet. Unfortunately, the message that she got was bariatric surgery was a quick fix, and she wasn't going to have to work on her eating habits. So, her first question after surgery is, "when can I have Doritos?"

I think the challenge that we have as we explore this topic is how are we going to get ourselves more centered in our approach to overweight and obesity? Let's start out with a few definitions. What is overweight? Overweight, defined as BMI standards, which we'll get to, "overweight" is a weight of between 25 and 29.9. Obesity is any weight BMI of greater than 30, so my little girl with her high BMI was clearly obese. We also have to use the word "overfat," and I know that's a sensitive subject, but we have to talk about people who are overfat. These are people who may have a normal BMI but are carrying more of their weight as body fat, and so that definition is overfat.

We know that obesity is now a global problem and it contributes to ill health, displacing undernutrition or malnutrition and infectious disease as the number one global nutrition-related problem. It is on the rise in every country in the world, in Southeast Asia, North Africa, and the Middle East, mostly in the industrialized areas. In the United States, the prevalence has increased over the last decade from about 25% to 66% of Americans fall into that category of overweight or obese. Unfortunately, children and adolescents are the group that's getting the biggest the fastest. One in six children and adolescents are overweight, and a similar number are at risk of being overweight.

I like to think about this way. If obesity was an infectious disease, like SARS or HIV, and we were looking at these gloom-and-doom statistics, as a country, we would marshal all of our resources in fighting this disease. Clearly, we're not there yet. The dichotomy here is that as obesity rates increase, we have an increased societal emphasis on thinness and weight management. Each year in this country, the diet industry makes between $40 billion and $50 billion from weight loss products. In the year 2000, a full 38% of adults were trying to lose weight. Unfortunately for most of us, insurance reimbursement for services is poor, and so most people are going to look for alternative ways of getting their weight under control.

Does dieting work? Clearly, it does. A recent study published in *The New England Journal of Medicine* suggests that any dietary strategy is going to work. But here's the caveat: You have to stick with it. Unfortunately, the average diet in the United States, when dieters have been surveyed, lasts two weeks. If I have 100 pounds to lose, two weeks probably isn't going to get me what I'm looking for.

There is more fraud and misinformation in this industry than any other. We're getting heavier, we're spending more money, but we're not getting the results. We know that children and adolescents are concerned with weight. In a study involving grade school girls, pay attention to this statistic, 28% to 40% reported being on a diet or concerned about being fat. We have this emphasis on weight. It's unpopular to be overweight, and we've got people dieting. But we're not getting the results. I believe part of it is also misinformation about the strategies to lose weight.

The YRBS data, and that stands for "Youth Risk Behavior Surveillance data," suggests that teens believe the best strategy to lose weight is to exercise and skip meals. Diet and calorie management doesn't rank as high. When you actually look at effective strategies, you have to have some caloric restriction. But surveys suggest that teens don't believe that.

Strategies. How do we get youth to understand this a bit better? There have been some suggestions that we need to post calories in schools and certainly in college dorms. If we post the calories of the meal for the day, will that be a good solution? The answer is no, it's not really a good solution. Harvard recently removed this information for fear of contributing to eating disorders because students were going in and selecting their foods based on the calories and not necessarily the nutritional value.

We've got to look at factors in the development of obesity. How did we get here? Obviously, there are biological factors, and as with every other chronic illness, genetics can rule the day. When both parents are morbidly obese, there's an 80% chance their children will be obese. That's a scary statistic. The good news is when neither parent is obese, there is less than a 10% chance their children will be obese. We've got this middle group. About 25% to 30% of obese people have normal weight parents, so where is the role of genetics?

Some great twin studies suggest that there is a genetic component. It's estimated that your genetic makeup can account for about 50%, up to 90%, of the variations that you might have in terms of your ability to store body fat. A way of looking at it is this: Genetics can load the gun, you can be behind the eight ball with this, but the environment pulls the trigger. You might have the genetic predisposition, but again, it's the environmental factors that may have the advantage of expressing those genes.

What about fat cells? Can we grow fat cells? What role do fat cells play in the development of obesity? Clearly, we have three different types of obesity that have been defined. We have hypercellular, too many cells; hypertrophic, big cells; and hyperplastic, many more cells. Hypercellular obesity is an above average number of fat cells. You can be born with them due to genetics, or you can develop them through overeating. Some older studies suggested that the number of fat cells that we had were fixed, and they just became bigger. Newer research is suggesting there's something else going on. You can also have hypertrophic obesity. These are fat cells that are larger than normal. These cells continue to expand as they fill with fat, and when they are full, the body now has the ability to make new fat cells. Here's the scary part: Once body fat is three to five times the normal amount, you generally have larger fat cells and you can make more of them, hyperplasia, making more cells.

Weight loss doesn't reduce the number of fat cells, making it difficult to lose weight once the body has created these fat cells. Why does this happen? When the fat cells become empty, biological triggers are signaled, saying, "you know what, I'm not happy with this. Eat more food. Fill me back up so I feel biologically normal." Sex and age are going to play a role in the development of obesity, and part of that is because males and females set different weight standards for themselves. Growth and development occurs at different rates and has a different outcome for boys versus girls.

I always say if I could rule the world, I would teach about puberty a little bit differently to adolescents than it is being taught now. Boys grow up and out under the influence of testosterone and add significant amounts of lean mass during puberty. Girls grow up and then they fill out. They add body fat under the influence of estrogen. That is a normal phenomenon. That should occur. That's the way it should be, but girls look at this as undesirable. They see their older brothers getting bigger and more muscular, and they look and say, "Okay, now I've got fat on the inside of my thighs. I've got a little fat on my tummy." That is absolutely normal; that is not pathology.

In childhood, boys are less likely to think they're overweight, and males in general are more accepting of personal weight gain. Well, that would make sense. If I'm gaining weight and I'm going to add a significant amount of lean mass, no wonder you'd be more accepting of personal weight gain. In early adulthood, the same number of men want to lose weight versus gain weight, where almost all women in early adulthood are looking to lose weight. Adult males tend to see themselves as overweight at higher weights, where women think they're overweight when they're closer to that healthy, ideal body weight. In fact, some studies suggest adult women only feel thin when they're about 10% below their ideal body weight. Therefore, we have this unbelievable difference in the way men and women view weight.

Both men and women gain most of their weight between the ages of 25 and 34, and for women, that weight gain can continue to go through menopause. There's been one study that suggested that most women from the ages of about 25 to 40 gain 20 pounds. It's this insidious weight creep that gets most of us.

There's a role of race and ethnicity in weight gain. We know American Indians, African Americans, and Hispanic women are more likely to be overweight than white women, but again, the rates are going to be similar for men. Black, Hispanic, Native Americans, and Pacific Islanders typically value thinness less than white Americans. I'm going to put it in a different context. I'm going to suggest that other ethnic groups, other than Caucasians, tend to have a more normalized view of what weight should be, not this distorted view of, "I need to be less than 100% of my ideal body weight."

We now know that there's an actual science of satiety, and remember, satiety is that feeling of fullness. This is under the control of two relatively newly discovered hormones, leptin and ghrelin. Leptin signals that the body has had enough food, so it's the off switch in terms of satiety. Leptin resistance, however, can occur like insulin resistance in diabetes. What does this mean? What that means is that you're producing leptin, but your body is not using it effectively, and you don't get that off switch. You might have read some studies in the newspapers suggesting that sleep deprivation may contribute to obesity. Leptin actually decreases with sleep deprivation. So that old adage of getting 8 to 10 hours of sleep per night really may be an effective weight loss strategy.

In the human body, we always have opposing hormones. In this case, ghrelin is the hormone that stimulates appetite. It's the on switch. I think in the years to come, we're going to see some pharmacology directed to manipulating those hormones, and that's a few years off.

Certainly, social and environmental factors can play a role in the development of obesity. Americans are more likely to be obese if they have a low socioeconomic status. Why is that the case? Oftentimes if you spend time, and I do, I'm very privileged to work in an inner-city high school in Houston, you see higher rates of obesity. But the reasons are many.

If you go around the high school that I'm at, there are no grocery stores. People would have to take a bus to go to the grocery store. It's the availability of grocery stores. It's the safety of neighborhoods. It's the quality of food that they can get. Certainly, when I leave the high school, where most of my teens are getting their food from is the convenience store down the street.

Well, we've all shopped at convenience stores, and that's what they are, they are convenient. They're not designed to give you all the rich produce that you can get in bigger grocery store chains. Poverty, also. Certainly, many individuals under the federal poverty line have very few resources in terms of putting together or constructing a healthier diet. Quite honestly, fat and sugar calories are unbelievably cheap.

We also see obesity rates rising among the affluent as well. The challenge we have, however, is we have a social stigma against individuals who are overweight. Employers, for example, want to hire people closer to ideal body weight. Now, is this bias or is it practicality? If you're an operating room nurse weighing 400 pounds, you might not be able to navigate around the OR table. Therefore, there is a space constraint there. What are we going to do? I think yes, employers want to hire individuals closer to ideal body weight, aesthetically, and then there's the practical side. Are some of our overweight clients and patients and employees going to be able to navigate around? Level of education is associated with body weight as well, but mostly only for women, illustrating the different standards for men versus women.

And then the media, my goodness, the media. We are bombarded with images of individuals who are lean and fit—in a country that's getting heavier. Again, we've got this wide divergence between individuals who are overweight and then are exposed to these media influences of ideal body weight. Certainly, in the last Olympics when some of the women competitors were heavier, disparaging remarks were being made about their body weight, but you didn't hear it about the men in the Olympics.

We can talk about the modeling industry, we can talk about beauty pageants, and we often see these weights creeping down in an overweight society. There have been some estimates that suggest that to be a Miss America, your percent ideal body weight needs to be 10% to 15% below ideal. We've got now all these biological factors. We've got environmental and social factors that are really complicating this.

One that doesn't get explored very often is something called the "built environment," and that influences our behaviors. For example, if you live in a neighborhood with no sidewalks, are you going to go out and walk? In my neighborhood, I can walk to the end of my road and then I'm right out on a busy street with very narrow sidewalks. I don't feel safe. I actually have to get in my car to go get physical activity. Think about inner-city neighborhoods. If you don't have walkability, including sidewalks, people are not going to be out and being physically active.

We have social factors as well in the way that we choose our food. We choose energy dense foods, lots of calories in a small space. As well, when we're with friends, we tend to overeat. Think about times that you've gone and spent time with relatives, and there's food everywhere. Someone says, "don't you want an extra serving?" or "You've lost weight in college. Let me fatten you up a little bit." Again, we've got these pressures to eat that oftentimes contribute to some of the social factors.

Science also suggests that we eat what's in front of us. If the portions that you're given are large, you tend to eat what's on your plate. Lifestyle and behavior factors as well. Physical activity comes up over and over and over again. But a lack of exercise is a major factor contributing to obesity. Only 22% of Americans get the recommended amount of exercise. Remember, that's generally somewhere in the range of 30 minutes a day most days of the week.

Here's something frightening: 25% of American adults are not active at all. All they do is go from their chair to the car, really not getting any kind of purposeful exercise. Television viewing is highly correlated with a low level of activity for both children and adults. For every two hours of television you watch, you can watch the rates of obesity rise. Why is that the case? Most of us are not terribly active while we're watching television. Here's a tip for you: Get an exercise bike, put it in front of the television, and make sure that you use that bike for at least 30 minutes of your television viewing a day.

Psychological factors. Do people over eat for other reasons besides hunger? Certainly. People eat to cope with stress, alleviate boredom. We have this category of restrained eaters that are really trying hard to control their weight. But they'll reduce their calorie intake by fasting or avoiding foods, and then overeat when stress triggers the release of that inhibition. This can occur when normal weight women perceive themselves as fat and are really trying to force their weight lower than biologically intended. Keep in mind habits can be passed down from mother to daughter. I am saying mother to daughter because it's more women who have restrained eating than men.

Think about this. If you come to the dinner table and you criticize the way you look or say, "boy, I've gained weight," your daughter or granddaughter sitting there listening to you now thinks this is what women do. Women have self-deprecating talk. They criticize the way they look. This is what normal women do. Now, people with healthier lifestyles, who communicate, manage conflict, manage problems better, often tend to manage their weight better as well.

We've got to get down to the nuts and bolts. How do we know if we're overweight? Well, BMI is the gold standard of population-based measurements of overweight. So if you're reading a study or you read something in the newspaper, 9 times out of 10, they are going to give you the BMI of that population. There are web-based ways of calculating your BMI. If you're Internet-savvy, www.cdc.gov provides a useful BMI calculator. If you like to crunch numbers a little bit, you can take your weight in pounds times 703 and divide by your height in inches squared. In general, a BMI of less than 24.9 is considered normal weight, so give yourself a pat on the back. If you're between 25 and 29.9, you're considered overweight. A BMI of greater than 30 is considered obese.

Remember, BMI is a population-based standard. It's not necessarily the best assessment tool for an individual. For example, athletes have a high BMI. In my world of professional football players, we encourage a high BMI. We're encouraging it because we want more muscle mass. Remember, muscle weighs something, so individuals who have an elevated muscle mass, their weight's higher on the scale, but their percent body fat can be lower. I think the challenge is BMI is not necessarily the best individual tool. Again, if you're very physically active, you might want another assessment technique.

Within that category of BMI, what it doesn't account for is individuals who are normal weight, BMI looks great, but they're metabolically obese.

Remember that woman who was five foot six inches and 118 pounds that we discussed? She was 40% body fat. She was normal weight, but metabolically has all the risk factors for someone who's overweight. Certainly, for most of us, BMI is going to be great. BMI can predict chronic risk of the big three—heart disease, diabetes, and cancer—because they all increase with increasing BMI.

The definitive assessment for body composition, if you are one of those outliers, is your percent body fat. My percent body fat can tell where in this range I am, so for example, say I have a normal BMI, but I want to see what that body composition is. How much of my weight is muscle versus fat? I can go get a percent body fat done. If a woman has a percent body fat of greater than 30%, or for a man greater than 20%, lo and behold, that can be a predictor. Where do you get this done? There are two different types of tests that you can get. One is called the "BOD POD," and we'll have more about this in your guidebook. The other is underwater weighing. Those are two things that you really have to go to an exercise facility to get done.

What about the health risks of being overweight or obese? One of the things we have to understand is the longer the obesity persists, the higher the risks. It is now presumed that the rising rates of obesity will reverse the actual increases in life expectancy that we've seen in this country. One of the great physicians I work with, Dr. Bill Klish, really brought this home to me when he said, children that are born in the year 2000 will be the first generation of children that don't outlive their parents. What's going to change life expectancy is going to be obesity.

Obesity-related diseases are costing the American taxpayers billions of dollars. What do we know? Overweight people are two to six times more likely to develop hypertension. They're more likely to have increased risk for stroke, deep vein thrombosis, clots in the legs. We know excess body fat can lead to impaired cardiac function from the increased mechanical workload on the heart, as well as just the heart not being able to pump as effectively. We know from previous lectures that abnormal amounts of blood fats and lipoproteins are associated with obesity, including high blood triglycerides, low HDL, and again, that high LDL/HDL ratio.

Excessive body fat can lead to insulin resistance and increase the likelihood of type 2 diabetes in both adults and children. We're going to cover this in more depth in the lecture on metabolic syndrome. Obesity can be an increased risk factor for the development of cancer because part of the eating patterns that get us to obesity, most people don't become obese by eating fruits and vegetables. Most people become obese by that increased amount of hidden fat and sugars in our diet, and certainly, those kind of dietary strategies are a risk factor for cancer.

Inactivity is also a cancer risk. In fact, some estimates suggest that poor diet and exercise may account for up to a third of the cancer risk. Excess body fat can lead to different types of cancers, most notably endometrial cancer, prostate cancer, colon cancer, and there's a thought about breast cancer as well. Obese people are more likely to have degenerative joint disease, osteoarthritis, and gout which is a deposition of painful uric acid crystals in the joint that makes it difficult to ambulate.

In the world of professional football, what contributes to obesity in retired football players is they have osteoarthritis from playing the game. They become obese. They develop gout. What do you think that does to your ability to ambulate and be physically active? It decreases it. That gout is oftentimes linked with insulin resistance, the inability to use your insulin effectively, comes up over and over again in terms of chronic disease risk.

Obese people are more likely to have sleep apnea, mechanical breathing constraints, particularly during exercise. It just takes more effort to work the chest wall if the chest wall has increased amounts of fat. Certainly, individuals who are overweight have more problems with anesthesia during surgery, as well as compromised wound healing. Other risk factors include gallbladder disease. Remember, that gallbladder is the storage house of bile, and when there's a lot of bile production, you can actually get an increased likelihood of gallstones.

A new and emerging consequence, however, is fatty infiltration of the liver. It is known as "nonalcoholic steatohepatitis." Some estimates suggest as that liver becomes infiltrated with fat, it causes hepatitis, and that hepatitis can actually lead to liver failure and transplantation.

Oftentimes, what's underestimated in this overweight and obesity is the psychological burden. Depression, being stigmatized by peers, bullying for children, discrimination. I call this the last accepted form of discrimination. We don't really have a great resolution. Certainly, we are sensitive to the fact that we have different religious beliefs and different cultural beliefs. We're different based on our ethnicity. We're sensitive to that, but we're not so sensitive to the individuals who are overweight. In terms of a public health initiative, obesity really needs to be the new smoking campaign. We need to get behind obesity like we did with cigarette smoking, and hopefully get the same kind of great results.

There are other costs that we see. In 2002, the cost of overweight in this country and obesity was estimated to be $92 billion. In a day of fiscal responsibility and all of us trying to tighten our belts, $92 billion being spent on obesity treatments, co-morbidities, disease.

There is good news. There is a silver lining here. Losing weight can reduce these disease biomarkers. People that are obese who lose as little as 5% to 10% of their body weight, just small amounts, can have improvement in blood pressure, improvement in insulin levels, glucose, cholesterol, and triglycerides. You don't have to lose 80 pounds to get good results. As little as 5% to 10% weight loss can help.

The perception of weight. Weight and the way we view weight is oftentimes dictated by what we see, the way the celebrity models can oftentimes give us what desirable weight is. But, keep in mind we don't have to get to that weight in order to have a desirable outcome. Just 5% to 10% of your body weight. Health-care professionals really do treat obesity like a disease, with multiple contributing factors. In the health-care world, we're going to emphasize health and fitness over necessarily what you should weigh on the scale. We're going to emphasize moderation and balanced diet, low fat, high in healthy foods, behavioral change as a process that requires really a new skill set that must be taught. If I always eat X when I get home from work in the afternoon, I'm going to have to work really hard to change that behavior if that X food is a high fat, high sugar treat. We're going to have to promote, as a health-care team, a substantial increase in moderate activity because keep in mind, a good percentage of Americans get no activity at all.

Frequently asked questions. What is weight cycling? I hear that all the time. What is this weight cycling phenomenon? Weight cycling is a pattern of losing and regaining weight over and over and over again. You hear people joke, "I've lost the same 100 pounds 10 times." What ends up happening is when you weight cycle, and particularly when you lose weight quickly, if you lose weight quickly, you're losing body fat and body muscle. When you regain the weight quickly, you're gaining back mostly body fat. Here's the problem. I'm losing metabolically active tissue when I diet, i.e. lean mass, and I'm regaining back more fat than I had before. What I'm doing with weight cycling over and over and over again is I'm dropping that functional lean mass, that wonderful metabolically active tissue, and I'm replacing it with just extra weight. The best example I can give you is Oprah. I admire her. She's unbelievably courageous. She gives us all of her weight struggles in a very public venue. But you see her struggle over and over and over again with weight cycling.

There are individuals out there in this anti-diet movement saying we should have size acceptance. What about these people? I do believe we need size acceptance in this country. We really have to have a different way that we're looking at obesity. I think, however, there's a downside to this size acceptance, which is that oftentimes we're not calling obesity what it is. It is a disease. If we think about it as a disease, we're going to treat the consequences. I think in treating the consequences, the co-morbidities, we have a better chance of doing that.

From a psychological standpoint, I'm going to tell you I think it's great. However, in terms of a physiological standpoint, I think the challenge is you can still have risks associated with that weight, and we do have to address those.

I appreciate everyone's attention through this weighty subject, and thank you very much.

Healthy Weight Management
Lecture 21

How do we affect weight change? Total energy intake, I've got to reduce how many calories I'm taking in, and I've got to change how many calories I'm expending.

One strategy to prevent overweight and obesity and manage a healthy weight is to adopt a healthy weight management lifestyle. The challenge for all of us is focusing in on a lifestyle that includes eating healthy foods, getting exercise, thinking positively about our food choices and our body image, and learning how to cope with stress. How many of us have been successful in managing our weight?

To affect weight change, we have to reduce total energy intake and increase total energy expenditure. Total energy intake is determined by the amount of calories you take in as carbohydrate, protein, and fat. Total energy expenditure is how many calories you burn and is determined by your basal metabolic rate, the thermic effect of food, and your physical activity level.

If you are trying to prevent weight gain, restricting your diet by just 200 to 300 calories a day will help you manage your weight in the long term.

Along this path of optimal wellness, we have to take a look at goal setting. First, aim for a body weight that optimizes your health—that at least prevents or stops weight gain—and aim for metabolic fitness. Focus in on a lifestyle that includes healthy foods, exercise, positive thinking about body image, and coping with stress. If you develop a lifestyle for successful weight management during early adulthood, healthy behavior patterns have a better chance of taking hold.

The most effective strategy for controlling your weight is managing your energy balance. If you are trying to prevent weight gain, restricting your diet by just 200 to 300 calories a day will help you manage your weight in the long term. MyPyramid.gov, an online tool, can help you balance your food intake. Overconsumption of food is always related to portion size. We have to realize that crash diets do not work.

How do I balance these energy sources? Fat intake should be lowered modestly to 20%–35% of your total daily calories. Carbohydrates should be between 45% and 65% of your total daily calories. In balancing energy sources, protein is a great way to eat something that is nutrient dense, but a diet that is higher in complex carbohydrates and moderate in protein is a better path to take. Protein should be in the range of about 10%–35% of your total calories.

The topic of eating habits gets us into more of the behaviors of food that are important to weight management. Physical activity is essential to weight management and promotes fitness and overall good health. Create a program that includes some kind of cardiorespiratory endurance as well as resistance training and stretching exercises. In addition, reframing the way we think about ourselves and our world by reducing stress and negativity will improve our behavior.

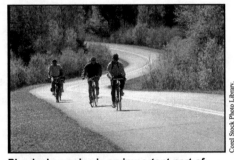

Corel Stock Photo Library.

Physical exercise is an important part of healthy weight management.

What do we know about life and long-term weight management success? For most individuals, initial success in weight loss relates poorly to their long-term success efforts. Physiologically, in addition to the changes in metabolism, there is a difference in fuel use, which affects your weight loss rate. When the weight loss slows, it means you are using more of your body fat as an energy source, so do not get discouraged. When weight loss plateaus occur, stick with your plan! Individuals who track their weight on the scale are more successful in the long term.

The American Dietetic Association lists 10 ways that you can cut calories. (Get the full list at American Dietetic Association, "Ten Ways.")

1. Get the facts—know what is in your food.

2. Limit alcohol.

3. Use smaller plates.

4. Order kid-size portions.

5. Serve in the kitchen; eat in the dining room.

6. Eat slowly.

7. Use plates—do not eat straight from the package or tray.

8. Eat plant foods—fruits, vegetables, and whole grains.

9. Switch to lower-fat dairy products.

10. Dull is better—food that appears shiny is likely high in calories.

What about individuals who struggle with being too thin? The causes are multifactorial: It can be an altered response to hunger and external cues including sense of time, distorted body image, metabolic and hereditary factors, prolonged stress, bizarre diet patterns or inadequate diets, or an underlying disease. To gain weight, they should eat small, frequent meals that are nutrient and energy dense; drink fluids at the end of the meal or between meals; use timers or other cues to prompt eating, and take a well-balanced vitamin and mineral supplement.

Exercise is still important, but they may want to do some isometric exercises or strength training to promote lean body mass gain and cut back a little bit on the aerobic activity. ∎

Suggested Reading

Brown, J., *Nutrition Now*, units 11–12.

Mahan and Stump, *Krause's Food, Nutrition, and Diet Therapy*, chap. 23.

Questions to Consider

1. Why are most weight problems considered lifestyle problems?

2. How do stress and other emotions affect your personal eating habits and food choices?

Healthy Weight Management
Lecture 21—Transcript

Welcome. How many of us have ever tried and been successful in managing our weight? I'll give you an example.

I was working with a very busy attorney in Houston and he had three law offices all around the country. His challenge was he was in the airport so much, and ate out so much, those were his barriers. What we worked on was getting him to be more active. Instead of him sitting down waiting for his plane, because he spent lots of time in the airport, we got him a pedometer and he counted how many steps he got in the airport. Then we changed the way he ordered from the restaurant menu. I'm happy to tell you he's now 36 pounds lower than he was in the past.

What we're really looking at here is how do we affect weight change? We have to really think about it as an equation. Total energy intake, I got to reduce how many calories I'm taking in, and I've got to change how many calories I'm expending. The example of my attorney is a great one to illustrate that point.

Total energy intake is actually determined by the amount of calories you take in, and it's composed of carbohydrate, protein, and fat. Total energy expenditure, how many calories you're actually burning, is determined by your basal metabolic rate, the thermic effect of food, and your physical activity level. Keep in mind this is a review on basal metabolic rate formula. First, you have to calculate your ideal body weight. So if I'm a man at 5 foot 10 inches, I would allow 106 pounds for the first five feet of height, and six pounds for every inch after. Therefore, roughly speaking, we're looking at between 1600 and 1700 calories for weight management. Along this path of optimal wellness, we have to take a look at goal-setting. How am I going to set my goal?

First and foremost, you should aim for a body weight that optimizes your health. Even though we've talked about an ideal body weight, that may not be a practical goal. How can I optimize my health? The first step is to prevent or stop weight gain. If you've been gaining weight on a regular fashion over the last couple of years, the goal is, can we stop that? Can we hold you steady in your tracks? You also want to aim for metabolic fitness, and this means that the biochemical risk factors, high blood pressure, triglycerides, all of those improve. Some science is going to suggest you can do that by losing somewhere in the range of 5% to 10% of your total body weight. Again, if I'm trying to lose 10% of my body weight, and say for example, my ideal body weight is 120, and I weight 200, even getting down to the range of about 180 pounds is going to help me to reduce my risk factors.

Then a challenge for all of us is we have to focus in on a lifestyle that includes eating healthy foods, getting exercise, thinking positively about our food choices, our body image, and learning how to cope with stress. Adopting this healthy weight management lifestyle is just that. Most of the weight problems we have are lifestyle problems. My attorney is an example. Very bright man, unbelievably successful, but he just wasn't able to negotiate around the barrier of travel and dining out. That's where I was able to step in and give him some guidance.

If you develop a lifestyle for successful weight management during early adulthood, healthy behavior patterns have a better chance of taking hold. You also need to adopt behaviors you can maintain. What might work best for me isn't what's going to work best for you, so you really have to look at what's going to be practical for me? What am I going to be able to do?

If we're looking at these dieting and eating habits, we've got to always, always address total calories. To lose weight, simple equation, you've got to take in fewer calories than you burn. Actually, the most effective strategy to control your weight is managing your energy balance.

If you're trying to prevent weight gain, restricting your diet just by 200 to 300 calories a day will long term help you to manage your weight. Now, there are tools out there to do that, and certainly, we want to focus on the balance of the food. There's a great tool online called "mypyramid.gov" that really can help you to balance your food intake. They actually have some weight management planners on there as well.

Overconsumption of food, as we've learned, is always going to be related to portion size. Most of us significantly underestimate the amount of food we take in. I will tell you, I have difficulty judging portion sizes and calories as well. I did a television interview in Houston where they asked me to go to some very popular Houston dining out experiences. They asked me to estimate the calories. It was a chicken fajita, no sour cream, no cheese, just meat, onions, and a tortilla, rice and beans. I came in and I had my books and my math, and I estimated that meal was about 1200 calories. As we actually analyzed that food, it was 1600 calories. When I say most of us significantly underestimate the amount of calories in food, that includes even health-care providers and including myself.

What we also have to do in terms of this healthy weight management is to realize crash diets don't work. These are diets that only contain minimum calories. And the example I always give is you can decide in your wisdom you're going to eat 500 calories. You can set that as a goal, and sooner or later, when the hunger kicks in, you're not going to be able to control it. Then we think, what's wrong with me? I should be able to make better choices. Why did I cave into the hunger? Why did I go eat that cookie? I liken that to sleep. I can set a plan that I'm only going to sleep two hours a night. Look at all the work I'd get gone. But the reality is, when the fatigue sets in and I fall asleep in front of the television, I probably wouldn't beat myself up the same way as I would if I overate on a very calorically restricted diet. As we look at crash diets, we have to balance that out with safer dietary approaches than some of the popular ones that are out there now, and we're going to cover that in a future lecture.

How do I balance these energy sources? Fat at nine calories a gram is going to be the easiest place for us to trim off those calories. You should avoid eating overly fatty foods. I think most of us know that. Fat is the most concentrated source of calories. If you limit the fat in your diet, it can help to limit your total calorie intake. Also, fat calories are more readily converted to body fat than calories from protein and carbohydrate. There's another good reason to do that. Fat intake should be lowered modestly to 20% to 35% of your total daily calories. High-fat, low-fiber diets tend to make us not feel very full and encourage overeating.

The trick is that foods that are labeled "low fat" or "fat free" can actually be high in calories. Despite lowering their fat content in order to make the food taste good, oftentimes what they do is increase the sugar. I remember when SnackWells cookies were popular years ago, and they were fat free. The message was if it was fat free, I could eat as many as I wanted. It's actually been termed the "SnackWell effect" because people just ate more cookies. Part of it is the fat makes the food taste good, and when I take that out, it doesn't have the same sensory experience as if I ate a real cookie.

Balancing energy sources should also include looking at the carbohydrate intake of your diet. Most authorities are going to suggest between 45% and 65% of your total daily calories should be based from carbohydrate. However, some people are going to do better with a reduced carbohydrate intake, and those are our friends who have insulin resistance. Avoid mixing these carbohydrate sources with high-fat toppings, and again, the best example is a baked potato. You take this lowly baked potato at 80 calories, you add all the stuff that you're going to pile onto it, and now you've got a potato that could be 300 or 400 calories.

High-sugar foods also are things you have got to be challenged with in this carbohydrate intake because they provide calories, but really few nutrients. The goal is, I want something that's nutrient dense, not energy dense. In balancing energy sources, protein is going to be a great way to do that, but that doesn't mean a high-protein/low-carbohydrate diet is going to help you. It doesn't conform to the dietary guidelines for Americans. It certainly isn't going to fit in the DASH diet for hypertension. The challenge is when I go to one extreme—instead of driving down the middle of the road, I'm trying to live in the ditch—eating an all-protein diet is not going to promote optimal wellness. I'm also going to suggest to you we're looking at a lifestyle modification. A diet that is higher in complex carbohydrates and moderate in protein is a better path to take. Protein helps to promote a sense of fullness. You have to be careful here because foods that are high in protein can also be high in fat. Protein should be in the range of about 10% to 35% of your total calories.

Eating habits. This really gets us into more of the behaviors of food that are important to weight management and some eating habits that work. The science will suggest eating small frequent meals on a regular schedule can work for many people. However, if you can't define "small," if the definition of a small meal is beyond your capabilities, I'm going to define it for you. A small frequent meal should be between 200 and 300 calories. If your small frequent meal is 600 to 700 calories, it's now turned into six large meals instead of six small meals.

Morning intake is really much more filling than late night eating and also tends to reduce overall energy intake. Think about this from a practical standpoint. If you're eating at night, are you generally having a bowl of cereal or a scrambled egg? Are you having a turkey sandwich? We tend to go for sweet or savory snacks late at night and, again, high calories, low nutrition. We know that skipping breakfast—and yes, you are right and your grandmother was right, breakfast is the most important meal of the day. We know that skipping breakfast can alter the way we use insulin. It can raise LDL cholesterol and total cholesterol. Often, skipping breakfast leads to higher energy intake later on in the day. If you skip breakfast and say, oh, I don't really have much of an appetite. I'm okay. Lunch comes, you eat lunch, and then all of a sudden, that hunger that was actually there kicks in. Three in the afternoon, you're starved and you go for a cookie or even an energy bar. You go and get a coffee drink with whipped cream, and now you've really exceeded your calorie intake for the day. No food needs to be entirely off limits and everything in moderation, but you have to eat breakfast.

Physical activity. Physical activity is essential to weight management and it promotes fitness and overall good health. It also has a really nice side benefit in that it discourages overeating by reducing stress and really produces some positive feelings of wellbeing. Most scientists will say it's because of the endorphin release that you get from physical activity. Now, the secret is if you're just trying to maintain weight and you're at an ideal weight, 30 minutes of moderately intense physically activity every day is good. If you need to lose weight, you probably need to aim for 60 minutes per day. I'm trying to create a calorie deficit.

How do I control or set up this exercise program? Create a program that includes some kind of cardio-respiratory endurance as well as resistance training and stretching exercises. Cardio exercise—walking, biking, I would put gardening in there—that you can sustain for about an hour can help to trim that body fat permanently. However, strength training can help to increase lean body mass which burns more calories at rest. It is more metabolically active than body fat. So the key would be I might want to go out and walk, garden. It doesn't have to be all at one time. I can certainly go out and take a 30-minute walk in the morning and I can ride the exercise bike at night. That might be a strategy to get those 60 minutes. Strength training, you want to concentrate on big muscle groups. You want to lift heavy enough weights where it becomes a bit of a challenge. I will always encourage you to take a look and talk to your physician or your primary health-care provider to make sure that you're physically able to do that kind of exercise.

In addition to creating this overall exercise program, you almost have to reframe the way you think about yourself and your world because that's going to influence how you feel and act. When we compare ourselves to that ideal self, we are more likely to have low self esteem. In a perfect world, I'd look the same way I did when I was 20 years old. That might be my ideal self in my mind. That's not going to be a realistic goal. If I strive to do that, I can end up not feeling great about myself. When you do that, you're setting perfectionist goals that are hard to attain. What you really want to do is replace that with really positive self talk, when you take yourself through the steps of a job and then praise yourself when it's successfully completed.

I'll give you an example. Say, for example, every afternoon, you're having a regular soda. Then you make a conscious effort, it's in your behavior plan, "I'm not going to do that any more. I'm really going to work on getting rid of that." Maybe for the next week, five out of seven days you've given that up. Don't concentrate on the two days you didn't do it. Concentrate on the five days that you did. That can be the opposite of that negative self talk. We make self-deprecating remarks or angry or guilty producing comments when you blame yourself unnecessarily. If you say, why did I do that? I have no self control. I have no self discipline. Realize that you're human and the reason why you do that is you haven't really explored, how can I manage my environment?

For example, if I'm a soda person, maybe the environmental management that I need to avoid the negative self talk is changing a behavior. You could say to yourself, you know, I'm not going to buy this. I'm not going to bring it into my house. So if I really have an urge to do that, I'm either going to have to stop on the way home or I'm going to have to go to a vending machine. I'm going to give myself just that minute to think about it.

We can also look in terms of changing our emotions and behaviors around food. We can also talk about stress management. How do I manage stress? Often, it's not a knowledge deficit that contributes to weight. It's, "I don't know how to environmentally control it." So we can look at one model, and this is the ABC model of behavior. It helps you to manage the events that trigger behaviors and factors that reinforce them. We have the "A," the antecedent: that event that precedes the behavior and might trigger it. Again, maybe it's a time thing for you. It's three o'clock in the afternoon. Maybe it's the weekends where you say, "Saturday's coming. I'm going to take that day off and I'm going to eat whatever I want." There's something that precedes it that triggers the "B," the behavior, and that follows with the consequences, the "C."

Unfortunately, sometimes this ABC model could be desirable, that you're doing something great, or undesirable. The consequences that occur have the greatest influence in terms of helping us to manage that. I think as we look at this, think of an example that might be personal to you. You have a fight with your spouse, you go into the pantry, and you get a cookie. Then you feel really guilty about that. I'm going to suggest replace the guilt, replace the consequence, with some positive self talk. You've now identified something that you can change. You can identify the cues that trigger the overeating, and that really is the first step to changing or avoiding these triggers.

You can manipulate the antecedents to promote positive behavior. You can say, "every single time I get in a fight with my spouse, I end up eating cookies." What you might do then is realize you're vulnerable during that period of time, and so you don't allow yourself to get so riled up in that discussion that you're going to trigger that behavior to go back to food. Positive consequences, and I would probably say positive rewards, can help to reinforce those new behaviors.

You can also use that in terms of your weight management. Say, for example, you're controlling your weight. Rather than rewarding yourself with food, you're going to say, "I'm going to reward myself by going out and going to a movie or I'm going to buy myself something new." Balancing this acceptance and change really means that you're accepting yourself for who you are and you're going to really work hard to improve your general life satisfaction. If you must diet, if you really need to lose a significant amount of weight, use a combination of exercise and avoid those very low calorie diets.

How do I set that goal? I'm modifying my behavior. Do I understand my triggers? Do I have a realistic weight goal? A realistic weight goal is between a half a pound to a pound a week. Now, I know what many of you are thinking. I have a lot of weight to lose. I don't want to wait that long. Well, my response to that is you didn't gain the weight in 15 minutes and you're not going to lose it in 15 minutes. So you really have to look at strategies and lifestyle management, rather than the quick fix.

What do we know about life and long-term weight management success? For most individuals, initial success in weight loss relates poorly to your long-term success efforts. How does that work? If everybody's dieting and everybody's on a fad diet, the likelihood of them keeping off that weight really isn't going to be very likely. It's often been said that between 90% and 95% of people who lose weight regain that weight later. That's because they're looking for a quick fix. This also highlights the difficulty of trying to maintain a low-calorie diet, particularly if that low-calorie diet is outside of the bounds of what you can tolerate or maintain.

Weight loss plateaus oftentimes are triggers to individuals. Think about that ABC model. Weight loss plateaus are oftentimes when your behavior changes and you think, "here I go again. Every time I go on a diet, I lose weight the first week, and lo and behold, I can't lose any the second. I'm just going to give up. I'm going to quit trying." Weight loss plateaus occur for a couple of reasons. One, your metabolism slows. If your calorie levels are too low, your body looks at that and says, wait a minute. There's not enough energy coming in, and it's going to lower the metabolic rate. This makes your diet increasingly less effective, despite your restricted caloric intake. As you lose weight, this is good news and bad news, you become more energy efficient and you require fewer calories to maintain your lower body weight.

You also have to understand a little bit of the physiology. In addition to the changes in metabolism, there's a difference in fuel use. During the first few days of a diet, your body is burning its limited carbohydrate stores and some lean mass. I want you to go back and remember. How many calories are there in a gram of protein? How many calories are there in a gram of carbohydrate? Four. It doesn't take very long to burn those calories off. Additionally, because lean mass, or muscle mass, is predominantly protein and water, if I lose a pound of muscle, the estimates are that there are about 2000 calories in a pound of lean mass, and 3500 calories in a pound of body fat. The challenge is, if I lose that lean mass, it takes me less time to burn 2000 calories than 3500 calories. And so lo and behold, what ends up happening?

In most weight loss science, it suggests that it takes you about three to five days to actually start burning body fat. Why don't I use my body fat first and hang onto my muscle mass? That's because your brain must have carbohydrate. In the short run, your brain can't use anything other than carbohydrate, so the challenge is your body's going to have to burn protein because that can be converted into carbohydrate. It's going to have to use its limited carbohydrate sources because obviously that's carbohydrate, and your body's going to have to have a time to adapt to using less carbohydrate for the central nervous system.

That weight loss plateau usually occurs about the second week, and that really is signaling, yes, you may have a decrease in your metabolic rate, but you're also now burning more fat than you are protein. The question I'm going to have is, how many of us celebrate that? How many of us say, oh great, I'm on week two of my weight management plan and I'm not losing as much weight as I did the first week. We don't celebrate that. I'm going to suggest you should. When the weight loss slows, it means you're using more of your body fat as an energy source. So again, don't get discouraged. Celebrate. I'm trying to reframe the way you think about this.

The key message here is when weight loss plateaus occur, stick with it. Part of this means you've got to weigh yourself every once in a while. I'm going to say you only weigh yourself once a week, but you have to do it. One of the biggest triggers for who's going to be successful long term are individuals who hop on the scale. If you hop on the scale two or three times a day, you're really only measuring changes in your fluid status, and I would really discourage you from doing this. To lose weight, you have to restrict those calories to about 500 calories less per day.

Again, some tips that we can have to cut calories and change behavior, both are important. I'm going to suggest that you're going to want to refer to the guidebook, but I'm going to walk you through some of the tips from the American Dietetic Association. They give you 10 easy ways that you can cut calories. First and foremost, get the facts. Foods that can seem surprisingly healthy can be loaded with calories and fat, so check out the nutrition facts panel on the label. Again, in terms of the weight management strategy, calories rule. Although nuts are unbelievably healthy for you, depending on the nut, 70% of the calories are coming from fat, so a cup of nuts can be as much as 600 calories. Great nutrition, but what I'm seeing now is a lot of people who are becoming increasingly heavier with healthy foods because as we talk about all the healthy foods that are out there, they tend to overdo those portions. Get the facts.

Limit alcohol. Although it's fat-free, alcohol contains about 70 calories per ounce, and that's goes, again, for many of the other sweet drinks. One glass of sweet tea and one eight-ounce glass of soda a day are 320 additional calories. I can eat about four medium apples for 320 calories. If I did this every day, this equates to over 116,000 extra calories. If this is above and beyond what I need for my energy balance, I can gain 30 pounds in a year. The key tip is: don't drink your calories. Chew your food. Don't drink your food.

Switch to smaller plates. If you have a regular-sized dinner plate, what does that mean? One of the strategies that you can do is just put your food on a smaller salad-sized plate. That way, you can reduce your portion sizes. When you go out to eat, order child-sized portions. You can get kid-sized popcorn at the movie theater without any butter. It has 150 calories. If you get the bucket, it can easily top 1000 calories. Keep in mind we tend to eat what's in front of us, so if I only order the smaller size, I can finish all that and not have any problem. If I order the larger size, I'm going to overdo every single time I go to the movies.

Another tip: Serve in the kitchen, eat in the dining room. If you bring your plate to the table already filled, you won't be tempted to pick from the serving bowls in front of you. I have to tell you, I'm a picker. I can easily pick myself into an entire meal, so that's a tip. Serve your plate in the kitchen. Don't bring the serving bowls to the table.

Eat slowly. This is hard for a lot of people. It's unbelievably hard for me. Put your fork down and take a sip of water in between bites. My strategy when I go to a restaurant with friends is I actually sit on my hands because that way, I'm not going to go grab something. I have to give myself that environmental cue, maybe I can eat something.

Use plates. Snacking from packages or picking out of a brownie tray, absolutely deadly. Your brain only remembers what it sees. If I decide I'm going to have a cookie, I make it an event. I put it on a plate. I sit down and enjoy it. I don't grab the cookie out of the pantry and just snack on it.

Over and over again, we're going to say fill up on plant foods. Fruits, vegetables, and whole grains take up stomach space. They take time to chew. They take time to eat. For every member in your family over the age of two, switch to lower-fat dairy products. Reduced-fat, low-fat or fat-free dairy products contain significantly fewer calories. If you just switch from drinking two glasses of 2% milk to skim, you're going to save 80 calories every day. Over a year, that represents almost 30,000 calories and that can represent, again, a significant change in weight.

Another tip: Make small permanent changes that you can live with. That can make all the difference in the world. Here's a small permanent change when you eat out. Dull is good. I'm not talking about being boring, not dull as in boring, but dull as in not shiny. When you see anything at a buffet or a salad bar, if it's shiny, it usually means that there's been a coating of vegetable oil that's been added to the vegetables. When you eat out, for example, say,

"I want you to grill my steak, chicken, fish, fill in the blank, dry." They can put a rub of spices on it, but you want them to grill it dry. If it comes to your table shiny, they could have easily poured 300 to 400 calories of butter onto that plate.

For my attorney, that was his major dieting strategy. Here's what he did when he went to a restaurant. Everything was ordered dry. At some of his restaurants in Houston, as well as Dallas and New York where he travelled frequently, we calculated that he was saving 400 calories a meal by just changing what he ordered. Additionally, what he would do is ask to have the smallest steak on the menu and then he always ordered a double order of vegetables. Since he had to entertain and eat out, and that was part of his job, this was a really good way of him doing that. He loved drinking wine, absolutely loved it. My suggestion was, buy the most expensive glass of wine that you can, get a really good bottle, really enjoy it, and savor the wine. But you don't feel like you need three or four glasses of wine. I can't tell you he went to zero, but he significantly cut his alcohol consumption. That, again, has translated into great weight loss for him.

What about the other side of the coin? What about individuals who struggle with being too thin? Again, I think the causes are multifactorial. It can be an altered response to hunger, appetite, and external cues. I have individuals who, if there wasn't a clock on the wall, would forget to eat. There are some people who have a distorted body image. They compulsively diet or over-exercise, and that's a different category. You can have metabolic and hereditary factors. Is everybody in your family lean? I describe it as the weight falls off of some people. They skip one meal and their metabolic rate is so high, they struggle.

Prolonged stress. Stress hormones can really influence your hunger and fullness response. Some other relatively significant problems, such as addiction to alcohol or drugs, can mask that appearance. Bizarre diet patterns or inadequate diets, and certainly, there can be an underlying disease because illness almost always speeds up metabolic rate.

What about people who are trying to gain weight? Small frequent meals, but what we're going to do is not only have nutrient dense, but energy dense foods.

This would be a great time to pull out the nuts. In fact, my favorite weight management strategy for individuals who need to gain weight is actually trail mix, a variety of different nuts, some dried fruits, and now you've got something with a lot of nutrition in a relatively small space, and a lot of energy in a small space.

Another tip for people who want to gain weight is drink fluids at the end of the meal or between meals to avoid filling themselves up. Individuals who need to gain weight may actually want to pull out the juices because again, the juice is going to leave your stomach quickly. It doesn't fill you up. Again, it can be a valuable source of calories.

I will also suggest individuals use timers or other cues to prompt eating. I had a very dear friend who had metastatic cancer, and we actually got her a sports watch, setting the timer to go off every 30 minutes. That was a cue to her that even if she didn't have the signal for hunger, she was actually hungry.

Take a well-balanced vitamin and mineral supplement to make sure you've got all your nutritional needs. Exercise is still important, but you may want to do some isometric exercises or some strength training to promote lean body mass gain and maybe cut back a little bit on the aerobic activity so you're not becoming a calorie-burning machine.

In summary, weight management becomes a lifelong strategy. By managing it lifelong, you're going to have the best strategy to prevent the tsunami of obesity that we're seeing in this country. Thank you very much.

Metabolic Syndrome and Type 2 Diabetes
Lecture 22

The estimates in the United States are about 47 million Americans have metabolic syndrome. It's not the occasional person that is affected. This is really a public health epidemic.

In the United States, we have seen an explosion in our girth and a corresponding significant increase in diseases like metabolic syndrome and type 2 diabetes. This lecture will explore the health-care tsunami that these diseases represent and the prevention and treatment of these disorders.

We are going to explore the intricacies of metabolic syndrome and type 2 diabetes. A patient came to me with uncontrolled diabetes and asked for a diet and exercise program. I discovered that his toe had gangrene, so the exercise program would have worsened his condition. Metabolic syndrome and type 2 diabetes are a complex set of disorders, so we have to be vigilant in our understanding and management of them.

Metabolic syndrome and type 2 diabetes are consequences of the way we eat and exercise. Many people believe metabolic syndrome is not a disease but a clustering of risk factors: an increase in blood sugar, undesirable changes in blood fats, an increase in blood pressure, and the accumulation of body fat (central obesity). They believe it is our early warning system for type 2 diabetes. The causes of metabolic syndrome include being genetically predisposed, having excessive insulin resistance, and being inactive. To prevent metabolic syndrome, you have to moderate your weight.

Type 2 diabetes is the most common form of diabetes. In type 2 diabetes, the body makes insulin but does not use it effectively. Type 2 diabetes is diagnosed in those with a fasting blood sugar of greater than 126 mg per deciliter or an oral glucose tolerance test of greater than 200. Other factors that can raise blood sugar include medications and illness. Type 2 diabetes is increasingly more common in children.

There are a few factors that can influence the development of type 2 diabetes. Type 2 diabetes is genetic. However, the environment must be conducive to its development.

There have been major studies that indicate that lifestyle changes can prevent diabetes. The most dominant is the Diabetes Prevention Program. Dietary factors include controlling calories and controlling the amount and type of fat and carbohydrate intake. Diets rich in whole grains, which have magnesium, and cereal fiber have been shown to reduce the incidence of diabetes. Iron and sodium nitrate in meat may worsen insulin resistance in type 2 diabetes. Vitamin D is anti-inflammatory, which improves type 2 diabetes. Coffee, both decaffeinated and regular, and light to moderate amounts of alcohol demonstrated a decrease in the incidence of diabetes. Avoid high glycemic index foods, including juices.

Diets rich in whole grains, which have magnesium, and cereal fiber have been shown to reduce the incidence of diabetes.

Type 2 diabetes in children is directly related to the increasing levels of obesity in children. Our youngest patient at Texas Children's Hospital is 4, and complications of type 2 diabetes start to occur 10 to 15 years after the diagnosis, so that will be in her teens or 20s. Complications include neuropathy, retinopathy, and nephropathy. The cost of care for those with diabetes in 2007 was 2.3 times higher than for those without diabetes; as type 2 diabetes becomes a predominant type of diabetes in youth, we can expect to incur greater costs.

Let's review some frequently asked questions. What is type 1 diabetes? In type 1 diabetes, individuals do not produce insulin because their beta cells are no longer functioning. They are on insulin for the rest of their lives.

Is there a best practice for people with metabolic syndrome or type 2 diabetes? Reducing carbohydrate is a good management strategy.

Besides pigment changes, are there any other symptoms of insulin resistance? Belly fat.

Does sugar cause diabetes? It does not cause diabetes, unless it is contributing to obesity.

Can herbal therapies be used to treat diabetes? There is some science to suggest that actual cinnamon can help lower blood sugar. The problem is we have no true standards for the purity, safety, and efficacy of dietary supplements in the United States.

Is there a cure for diabetes? I do not think you can call it a cure in the medical sense, but if I can control all the comorbidities nutritionally, I would consider that a cure.

How do I combine all these dietary recommendations? The diets we recommend in this course are not so different; they all talk about controlling weight and exercise. In tweaking the DASH diet for those with metabolic syndrome, the key is reducing the carbohydrate even lower. A registered dietician can come up with the best plan for you. ■

Suggested Reading

Mahan and Stump, *Krause's Food, Nutrition, and Diet Therapy*, chap. 34.

McArdle, Katch, and Katch, *Exercise Physiology*, chap. 20.

Questions to Consider

1. Do you believe you or any members of your family are at risk for metabolic syndrome? If so, have you seen your health-care professional to discuss strategies for dealing with that risk?

2. What is the difference between type 1 and type 2 diabetes? How are they similar?

Metabolic Syndrome and Type 2 Diabetes
Lecture 22—Transcript

Welcome back. In this lecture, we're going to explore the intricacies of metabolic syndrome and type 2 diabetes. I'll give you an example of the severity of this illness. I had a man who came into clinic to see me who was referred by his physician because his blood sugars were really high and he had uncontrolled diabetes. We were sitting there, visiting a little bit, and in addition to being a dietician, I'm a diabetes educator. He said, well, the doctor said you're going to give me a diet to follow and an exercise program. I had the forethought to say, I wonder if anybody has ever checked this man's feet. So I asked him to take off his shoes, and actually, he had gangrene of his baby toe. Therefore, had I recommended an exercise program for him, I would have made his condition worse. Because this is such a complex set of disorders, metabolic syndrome and type 2 diabetes, we have to be really vigilant in our understanding, as well as management.

As Americans, we've seen an explosion in our girth and this is partly due to our affluent society. Metabolic syndrome and type 2 diabetes are consequences of the way we eat and the way we manage our exercise programs. Many people believe metabolic syndrome is actually not a disease but a clustering of risk factors. The risk factors for metabolic syndrome include an increase in blood sugar, maybe not high enough to have diabetes, undesirable changes in blood fats that we've explored in other lectures, most notably, an increase in triglycerides and a decrease in HDL, an increase in blood pressure, and the accumulation of what's called "visceral" or "belly fat." We've explored ways that you can figure out your own risk.

Other people will say, you know what, it's not really disease, so what is it? Many people believe it's our early warning system; our radar system that type 2 diabetes is on the way. Certainly, the Centers for Disease Control cite the Third National Health and Nutrition Examination Survey, sometimes abbreviated "NHANES," that says that the estimates in the United States are about 47 million Americans have metabolic syndrome. It's not the occasional person that is affected. This is really a public health epidemic. Also, the CDC estimates that 24 million Americans have type 2 diabetes, and many experts believe this is really under-diagnosed.

This lecture is going to look at the tidal wave that we have that these diseases represent, and the prevention and the treatment of these all-too-common disorders. What are the causes of metabolic syndrome? Like everything else, we can be genetically predisposed. We certainly know that individuals who have that central obesity, that apple shape, can really influence the development or maybe it's an early warning sign. Again, referring to your guidebook, we have ways of you calculating that.

The fat cells in abdominal or visceral fat behave badly. They don't behave like other body fat, and they actually increase the level of inflammation in the body. In the Jupiter study that we've referred to in the past, we know that individuals that have an inflammatory response, even if their LDL cholesterol, their "bad" cholesterol, is within a normal range, are at an increased risk of heart disease. So these badly behaving fat cells that increase inflammation really do have a significant disease risk associated with them.

Excessive insulin resistance. We've talked about insulin in the past, but how do you know if you have insulin resistance? First and foremost, you can look at where your body fat is stored. Secondly, you can look for something called "acanthosis nigricans." What this actually is is excessive pigment where the skin bends, where the skin can fold back. So you can see it on knuckles, most commonly you see it around the neck. You can see it under breast tissue, under fat folds, and it's a hyperpigmentation. It's not a hygiene issue. Actually, it looks like ring around the collar, so you see this hyperpigmented area around the neck.

I had a young lady who came into clinic. She had metabolic syndrome. She had acanthosis nigricans and she thought, "I'm just not cleaning myself well enough." She actually took a Brillo pad to her neck and tried to scrub off the pigment. It's pigment. It's not dirt. And why do we end up with this hyperpigmented area? Insulin, that wonderful anabolic hormone, stimulates the melanocytes, the pigment-producing cells, to make more color. If you're a person of color, if you're African American or Hispanic, it really looks like a dark or black ring around the collar. In lighter-skinned individuals, it can almost look like a brown discoloration, most predominantly on the back of your neck.

Are there any other things that we should be concerned about in terms of this metabolic syndrome? What else is going to cause it? Inactivity is the recurrent theme. Bodies are designed to move. The American College of Sports Medicine, in its wisdom, has come up with a campaign called "Exercise is Medicine." They want every physician in the United States to be comfortable in terms of writing an exercise prescription. Estimates vary, but most experts will say that the beneficial effects of exercise in the prevention and management of metabolic syndrome and type 2 diabetes last between 19 and 24 hours. So what that means is you need exercise every day if you either have metabolic syndrome or type 2 diabetes, or if you're at risk. Inactivity, in itself, makes the cells more resistant to the effects of insulin. Remember, the body has to crank out more and more and more of this wonderful anabolic hormone, and again, too much of a good thing in this case is not a good thing.

How do we prevent metabolic syndrome? Key themes: You've got to have a moderation of your weight. This is an example where you must, must, must exercise every single day. I want you to think about that as being as important as taking high blood pressure medication, as important as taking your statin resin if you have high cholesterol or any other medication that you're prescribed. I want you to start to reframe the way you think. Exercise is as effective as medication, so I must take it every day.

Choose this wonderful anti-inflammatory diet. The Mediterranean diet, which has a lot of vegetables, monounsaturated fats, nuts, seeds, olive oil, all are important. Don't ever step over the need to control calories. Calories are really important. And as we explored in the lecture on carbohydrate, the value of choosing carbohydrates based on their glycemic index. And again, whole grains being rich in magnesium are all pretty essential.

Type 2 diabetes. It is the most common form of diabetes, and again, estimates vary, but between 80% and 90% of diabetes is this type. What is type 2 diabetes exactly? It can be diagnosed by your physician and there are diagnostic criteria. In this case, the body makes insulin, but it's not being effectively used by the body. It's not an insulin deficiency here, at least in the early stages. It's not insulin deficiency; it's inappropriate use of insulin by the body. This is diagnosed by having a fasting blood sugar—you've had nothing to eat—of greater than 126 milligrams per deciliter, or an oral glucose tolerance test of greater than 200. But like with most metabolic parameters, over the last 20 years, we've seen numbers drop. When I first started in practice, diabetes wasn't diagnosed until you had a fasting blood sugar of greater than 140, so stay tuned. You're going to see these targets probably decrease in the next five or six years.

Other factors that can raise blood sugar are oftentimes not accounted for. We don't think about them. First and foremost, medications can raise blood sugar, and they can actually interfere with an appropriate diagnosis. Some high blood pressure medications can cause your blood sugar to be high. Niacin for high cholesterol, this is one of the reasons why you don't want to take niacin unless a physician knows you're taking it. Steroids, including steroids that you're using to control an illness, can affect blood sugar. If you're taking estrogen or testosterone, your blood sugars can be higher. An anti-seizure medication Dilantin can also raise blood sugar. So there are lots of other factors that can complicate or give an inappropriate diagnosis. You can imagine if you're taking niacin on your own, and you are at risk of developing diabetes, and now you go in and your blood sugar is high, then you're going to get an inappropriate diagnosis that was actually medication-induced.

Illness will raise your blood sugar. Fever raises your blood sugar. So what that means is independent of food, physical stress, not the emotional stress of a challenging job, but physical stress, or an insult to the body, can raise blood sugar independent of food. Well, a lot of people refer to type 2 diabetes as "adult-onset." What I hear more often in my clinical practice is, "you know, it's not a problem. I've just got a little bit of sugar." I'm going to try and raise the bar on that and get you to think about it in a different way. Although we think of type 2 diabetes, or adult-onset, as less dangerous, it's actually now being increasingly more common in children. Estimates are going to vary here, but the complications of diabetes are estimated to occur 10 to 15 years after diagnosis. I want you to think about that when we explore children and type 2 diabetes.

Historically, the type of diabetes that we've seen in children is type 1. This type of diabetes is insulin-requiring. They must have insulin to survive.

However, recent estimates from the CDC suggest that type 2 diabetes now accounts for between 8% and 46%, big range there, of all new cases of diabetes. Part of the difference in the range is how old that study was. What was the target at the time, was it 140 for a fasting blood sugar or 126? The most important take-home message is many experts now believe that prevalence is underestimated. Part of that is the signs and symptoms of diabetes are not things that are going to get your immediate attention.

In type 2 diabetes, is it in your genes? The recurrent theme is absolutely. Twin studies give us the best look at the genetics of diabetes. If you're an identical twin, you share an identical gene pool. If one twin gets diabetes, the chance that the other twin gets diabetes is three out of four, so you have a significantly greater risk. We now have identified multiple different genes, loci on genes, that will suggest that, yes, there are some higher risk individuals. However, the environment must be conducive to the development of type 2 diabetes. Estimates vary using CDC data, but the Pima Indians are an ethnic group with a prevalence of diabetes that's estimated to be about 50 out of 1000 subjects. A relatively high prevalence. Ethnically, Pima Indians rarely marry outside of their genetic gene pool, so they tend to preserve their gene pool.

A great example is diabetes in the Rio Grande Valley. One of the highest prevalence in the United States is down in the Rio Grande Valley down in Starr County. Part of that is the influence of the Pima Indian gene pool. We know we have a really high genetic component here in type 2 diabetes. Again, the Human Genome Project has identified over 17 genetic loci strongly associated with type 2 diabetes. It's the marker on the gene.

Does the environment contribute to diabetes? The clear answer is yes, that jury is in. Genetics can be against you. However, I want you to think about I've got this genetic susceptibility, but I do have the ability to control my environment and prevent it. I used to say we're all going to get something. If I know genetically I'm set up for diabetes, now I can get myself loaded. I can get myself ready to go. I bring out all my tools to prevent diabetes. But the great news for us is there have been some major prevention studies that indicate lifestyle changes, even in the face of genetic susceptibility, can prevent diabetes.

Probably the most predominant one is something called the "Diabetes Prevention Program." They assigned people, participants, with blood sugars that were just below the level of pre-diabetes to one of three groups: placebo, standard care; Metformin, which is a medication that is used to control diabetes; or lifestyle intervention. The lifestyle intervention included two-and-a-half-hours per week of physical activity—overall that's not going to be a huge amount of activity—and a healthier low–fat, low-calorie diet. Also this intervention was actually delivered by registered dieticians, and so there was some education as well. Lifestyle intervention, and to me, this is the "aha moment," reduced the incidence of diabetes by 58%, where traditional pharmacology that is used for the same kind of circumstances reduced it by 31%. It's not that it was reduced to nothing, but lifestyle ruled the day.

The weight reduction in the lifestyle intervention group, as initial weight loss was 7%. After almost three years of follow-up, the total weight loss was about 5%, so they did regain weight. However, they still had a significant reduction in the development of type 2 diabetes. A key message here is even if you can't lose a substantial amount of weight, any weight loss matters. If you have a family history of diabetes, or if you have metabolic syndrome, this is really great news.

Other dietary factors. Diabetes control is more than just controlling calories. The type of fat can influence diabetes in genetically susceptible individuals. Studies such as the National Nurses Study, which will also be mentioned in the lecture on heart disease, was a long-term study taking a look at a large number of subjects, and that gives science the best look at long-term risk factors. Those who had the highest trans fat intake had a much greater risk of developing diabetes than those who had a lower intake. There's a possible link between trans fats and inflammation, so think of that Jupiter study.

Those who had the highest intake of polyunsaturated fats, omega-6 and omega-3, had a decreased risk of developing diabetes, so the type of fat matters. However, when we look at poor intake of omega-3 fatty acids, when you don't have a good balance between those two major types of essential fatty acids, poor intake of omega-3 fatty acids, have been linked with insulin resistance. Keep in mind you want a nice balance.

The amount and type of carbohydrate can influence the development of disease. Diets rich in whole grains and cereal fiber have been shown to reduce the incidence of diabetes. What's our case for fiber? Those soluble gumming fibers make food leave your stomach slowly and you get a slow postprandial, after-meal, rise in blood sugar, so your body doesn't have to work as hard. It doesn't have to produce as much insulin to metabolize those sugars.

Magnesium that's found in whole grains. Some research suggests that magnesium may be the missing link between whole grains and diabetes. Could it be that it's really the magnesium content that's lost in the processing of the food that really helps to protect our bodies from the development of type 2 diabetes? Certain studies have shown that increasing the intake of whole grains can decrease the risk of diabetes by 40%. I want you to think about that for a second. That simple switch of buying a different type of bread, or a different type of breakfast cereal, particularly if you're genetically behind the eight ball, this is a really great strategy.

Other protective compounds include the glycemic index. Certainly, if you review the lecture on carbohydrates, we know that individuals that have a high glycemic index diet can actually increase the workload of the beta cell. And the beta cell is part of the body that makes insulin. This eventually can contribute to beta cell fatigue. The beta cells just can't keep up with that environmental demand.

Is there anything else? Well, the answer is absolutely yes. Iron. We know or we've heard of the word antioxidant, and we think of antioxidants as being good things. Iron is an oxidant. Iron may actually worsen insulin resistance in type 2 diabetes. Now, I have to tell you there's not a real clear answer here. Is it the iron or is it the meat? In the Iowa Women's Health Study, a relationship emerged between haem iron, this special kind of iron is only found in meat, and an increasing risk of diabetes. Again, I want to remind you, when we talk about controlling the portion sizes of meat like we did in the DASH diet, there's a reason beyond hypertension and there may be a link between haem iron found in meat and diabetes.

The association was stronger in this study in those who consumed alcohol. Iron overload is actually thought to contribute to damage to the beta cells. I have to tell you in my world of professional football, I see many athletes who have iron overload because we have so many fortified foods. We also know that the type of meat, particularly if it's processed with sodium nitrate, may also contribute to the damage to the beta cells. Again, plants tend to rule the day, and in this case, excess amounts of highly processed meat with sodium nitrate can actually damage the beta cells.

Eating meats with nitrates almost every day, and where do those come from? Well, think bacon, ham, bologna, had a greater than 40% chance of developing diabetes. Dose is everything. Most of us don't think of dose when we talk about meat, but I'm going to suggest to you that the American diet has more animal protein than it needs, and here's a good reason to try vegetarian. Certainly, in the Women's Health Initiative, there's been found to be a relationship between vitamin D and the development of diabetes. Part of the problem was they didn't really find a protective effect with vitamin D, and the problem was the dose probably wasn't high enough. A lot of estimates are out there now that our current recommended amount of 400 International Units is not enough to keep blood levels normal. Other studies suggest that, yes, vitamin D in a higher dose is protective against the development of both type 2 and type 1 diabetes.

Vitamin D, in and of itself, is anti-inflammatory, and it reduces insulin resistance. Here's the hard part, though. If I am overfat, vitamin D is actually sequestered or stored in body fat, making it less biologically available. So I'm consuming the vitamin D, it gets stuck in my body fat and it's not available to the blood. The beta cell itself, that insulin-secreting cell in your pancreas, is a direct consumer of vitamin D. It can convert it to its most active form. Again, the beta cell really relies on vitamin D.

What about beverages and diabetes? Coffee, you're not hearing caffeine here, nor are you hearing energy drinks, but we're talking here again about a whole food. Coffee, both decaf and regular, is associated with a decrease in diabetes. Again, this is a dose-related phenomenon. Increasing consumption from one cup to three cups provides some additional risk reduction. A great review of coffee consumption was in the *Journal of the American Medical*

Association in 2005, and it concluded that regular coffee consumption can substantially reduce the risk of type 2 diabetes. So now when someone questions how much coffee that you're drinking, you can be relatively smug and say, "I'm on my type 2 diabetes prevention program." Coffee is a very rich source of antioxidants, and actually outperformed tea, which really had no effect, another great reason to have that sugar-free, non-fat, decaf latte. You're getting some vitamin D. You're getting some calcium, and again, you're getting those rich antioxidants.

What about alcohol? The Physicians' Health Study indicated that for those consuming light to moderate amounts of alcohol, which we've defined, there was a subsequent decrease in the incidence of diabetes. It may not be the alcohol per se, but the antioxidants that are found in alcohol. Alcohol can actually reduce the production of glucose by the liver. But if you have diabetes, or you're taking medications for diabetes, always check with your physician to see whether or not alcohol is going to be part of your diet.

Let's think about this: What about sugared drinks? Now we have a double whammy here. Beverages don't promote satiety or fullness, like salads do. High glycemic index foods, which include juices, are probably something that you want to avoid. This includes soft drinks, sweet tea, lemonade, and fruit punch.

As we switch gears and talk about type 2 diabetes in children, I'm going to tell you this is a relatively new and for me, as both a clinical dietician and a diabetes educator, it's relatively disturbing to me. This is directly related to the increasing levels of obesity in children. I work in Houston. We have a very high Hispanic population. We know that African Americans and Hispanics have that genetic predisposition. But it's been estimated that close to 600,000 youths in the United States have some degree of glucose intolerance, and the incidence of type 2 diabetes has significantly increased in the last 15 years. Since I've been a dietician for 30 years, I have to tell you in my first employment at Tulane Medical Center in New Orleans, I never saw a child with type 2 diabetes. Now at Texas Children's, our diabetes clinic sees more children with type 2 diabetes than type 1.

Our youngest patient is four, so I'm going to remind you to think the complications of type 2 diabetes start to occur 10 to 15 years after the diagnosis. What does that mean for our youngest patient? The complications are going to occur for her in her teens or 20s. What kind of complications do we see? We see this general classification of what I call "opathies," a disease state. Neuropathy, issues with the nerves; retinopathy, issues with the eyes; nephropathy, kidney. Remember my man who had the gangrene in his toe? You might have been thinking, why didn't he feel that? Why didn't he have pain? He had significant neuropathy, where he couldn't feel his feet, so he didn't know he had gangrene. He had enough abdominal fat where he couldn't see his toes. Therefore, a strategy always is if you have type 2 diabetes, please, please, please check your feet because again, if I can't feel the pain, I've lost that ability to have my early warning system.

What about the economic cost of diabetes? Can we afford it from a population standpoint? According to the American Diabetes Association, the cost of care for those with diabetes in 2007 was 2.3 times higher than for those without diabetes. As we all struggle with controlling health-care costs, it would be wonderful if we actually paid for prevention. We don't pay for prevention usually in this country, and so what we're ending up doing is paying for it on the backside. As type 2 diabetes becomes a predominant type of diabetes in youth, we can expect to incur greater costs.

Remember, there's another type of diabetes. What about type 1 diabetes? It's similar in the fact that blood sugars are high, but it's different. In type 1 diabetes, the individual ends up producing no insulin. Their beta cells are not functioning any longer. They are going to be obligated to take insulin for the rest of their life. Most people believe it's an autoimmune disorder, and certainly, there are things called "diabetes seasons," where you actually see more diabetes being diagnosed in the winter month, cold and flu, than other times during the year. But it's represented by the ultimate destruction of the beta cell, so the cells of your body that make insulin can't make insulin any more.

Individuals that have type 1 diabetes are on insulin for the rest of their life. At this point, there's no other option. Certainly, in the future, we'll look at stem cell transplants, beta cell transplants and ways of seeing if we can control or correct type 1 diabetes. These patients are usually lean and usually young. Now, we certainly do know that many people can develop type 1 diabetes really at any time during their life, and so you've got to be on the lookout. Usually in people who are developing type 1 diabetes, because they've lost their anabolic hormone, they lose weight very quickly at the early stages of their diagnosis.

Is there going to be a best case scenario for people with metabolic syndrome or type 2 diabetes? I'm going to suggest to you the answer is yes. The reason is if indeed type 2 diabetes is you know what, I'm resistant to my own insulin. Insulin's an anabolic hormone. It promotes the deposition of body fat. What's the biggest trigger, what's the foot on the gas pedal for insulin secretion? The foot on the gas pedal is carbohydrate. Carbohydrate stimulates insulin production more than protein and certainly more than fat. This would be an example of taking a lot of the great public health guidelines, say anywhere between 45% and 65% of your diet should be carbohydrate, this is where you would modify it. If the biggest gas on the pedal is carbohydrate, this might be an individual where I'll take the carbohydrate lower than 45%. I've actually taken it down to as low as 30% in individuals that I just couldn't get the metabolic parameters to fall into place.

I'm going to say reducing carbohydrate in individuals with metabolic syndrome, type 2 diabetes, really is a good management strategy. Not zero carbohydrate, but reduced carbohydrate. You can also understand that the type of carbohydrate would need to be low glycemic, whole grain, and getting carbohydrates from healthy choices, and not necessarily the processed carbohydrates.

Another question I get all the time, other than these pigment changes, are there any other symptoms of insulin resistance? The answer is yes, it's that belly fat. It's that big belly that we've all seen. Hopefully none of us have that, but just in case, that big belly that we've all seen, that again is an outward sign that not only are you storing body fat, but that type of body fat doesn't behave itself. It's a more inflammatory body fat, and again, inflammation and insulin resistance go hand in hand.

Another unbelievably common question: Does sugar cause diabetes? The answer really is no, it doesn't cause diabetes, unless it's contributing to obesity. Sugar in and of itself in a lean individual is not going to cause type 2 diabetes. Sugar does not cause type 1 diabetes. Type 1 diabetes is an autoimmune disorder, and so there should be no guilt. "Oh my goodness, I drank sodas when I was 10 and that's the reason why I've got type 2 diabetes." That's not true.

I've heard there are herbal therapies that can be used to treat diabetes. This answer is actually a yes and a no. There is some science to suggest that actual cinnamon can help to lower blood sugar. The problem is, if I take cinnamon as a supplement, we have no true standards for the purity, safety, and efficacy of dietary supplements in the United States. Tragic in many instances. So I can go to the science and say, yes, there are science studies out there that suggest cinnamon is an effective strategy. The question is what brand am I going to recommend? If you're going to take it as a pill, is there a brand that I can guarantee? Unfortunately, no. If you like cinnamon in your sugar-free oatmeal in the morning, and you really like cinnamon added to different foods, by all means. The challenge is when you're talking about herbal therapies to treat diabetes or any chronic illness, it's generally more of the herb than you would ever naturally get in your diet. The challenge is, I can't get this and like my food, so the reality is many herbal therapies are going to fall short.

Is there a cure, because everybody wants a cure? I will tell you that I don't think you can say cure. Your insurance company's not going to say cure. Your physician might not even say cure. But I think from the Diabetes Prevention Study, I think what we can learn is that if I can control all the co-morbidities, if I can control the hypertension, and all the things that lead to poor outcome, I would consider that a cure. I'm going to consider that a cure. I've seen individuals whose blood sugars have normalized, their lipids have normalized, and their blood pressure has normalized, by losing weight and exercising and following some of the other dietary recommendations. Again, in the medical world, they probably wouldn't call that a cure. In the nutritional world, I'm going to tell you I would.

Another question: Will the DASH diet help to prevent metabolic syndrome or is it only meant to treat high blood pressure? How do I combine all these dietary recommendations? I think that's the bigger question. Does the diet from the American Cancer Society, the DASH diet, the diet from the American Diabetes Association, are they all that different? The answer really is no. They share some common themes. You're always going to hear controlling weight, you're always going to hear exercise, but the key is we can tweak it a little bit for our individuals with metabolic syndrome. Again, my strategy is I'll reduce the carbohydrate probably lower than the DASH diet would recommend because I'm trying to treat all of that. That would be a really good time to go see a registered dietician so they could assess your own risks and come up with the best plan for you.

Thank you very much.

Dietary Approaches to Weight Management
Lecture 23

We're going to take a look at individuals who are successful losers, using data from the National Weight Control Registry. ... so you can become a better consumer and better informed.

Research has found that moderately reducing food intake produces greater fat loss relative to the energy deficit. However, in a world where consumers want results yesterday, fad diets, pills, and supplements promise quick and easy fixes. This lecture will explain and critique some of the popular diets that exist today, as well as discuss methods for successful long-term weight management. Let's look at appropriate weight management strategies. We are going to take a look at what successful losers do and critique and explain some of today's popular diets.

The National Weight Control Registry gives us information on what successful losers do. They eat breakfast every day, weigh themselves at least once a week, exercise for approximately an hour every day, reduce their amount of television time to less than 10 hours per week, and they restrict calories and often follow a low-fat diet. How can you tackle this strategy of weight management? You can get self-help books and manuals, use meal replacements, join self-help groups or go to a private counselor, physician, psychotherapist, or registered dietician. There are also commercial programs such as Jenny Craig and Nutrisystem.

In a world where consumers want results yesterday, fad diets, pills, and supplements promise quick and easy fixes.

The most popular and most controversial diet over the last 30 years has been the Atkins diet. It is a low-carbohydrate, ketogenic diet that says you can eat whatever you want as long as it is just from protein-containing foods. The success of this diet comes from the fact that when most people limit the amount of carbohydrate, they end up decreasing their total calorie intake due to taste fatigue. The initial weight loss is largely due to dehydration, which does not necessarily reduce your body fat. Low-carbohydrate diets can also cause a significant reduction in lean mass, which reduces your basal metabolic rate.

This diet remains credible to some because you can see some improvement in health. The Atkins diet needs more long-term research on overall health risks.

When would you use a very low-calorie diet, something under 1000 calories a day? Individuals that have severe clinical obesity may be candidates for one of these programs. Advocates of these programs will suggest your limiting your daily calorie intake to between 400 and 800 calories of mostly high-quality, protein-containing foods. The most popular version is Medifast.

If we do not want to do the dieting extreme, what else can we do? Weight Watchers is probably one of the most successful commercial programs out there because it contains all the components of a successful diet. The South Beach diet was written by a cardiologist and is low-glycemic focused. Exercise is not a popular or effective "diet," but it prevents weight regain.

Over-the-counter drugs and dietary supplements for weight loss contain caffeine, benzocaine, or fiber. Ephedra helps with short-term weight loss, but it is dangerous in people with hypertension, heart disease, or diabetes. Two antiobesity drugs are approved by the FDA: Meridia, an appetite suppressant, and Xenical, which interferes with fat digestion and absorption. The benefits of drug therapy over behavioral modification interventions are modest at best—most people, although they will lose weight, cannot live on amphetamines.

The last resort is surgery, and it can be effective in individuals who have morbid obesity—a body mass index of greater than 40. Gastric banding reduces the size of the stomach by creating a smaller upper stomach, allowing smaller intake. Gastric bypass reroutes some of the small intestine so that it malabsorbs some calories. The results with gastric bypass or gastric banding are that patients lose substantially more weight in the initial phases; however, the weight loss tends to plateau. The long-term effectiveness of this program depends on how people manage their eating.

What does work? Decrease your energy intake by 500 to 1000 calories below daily expenditure by moderately restricting food intake. Keep tabs on your habits and become involved in activities other than eating, especially fitness activities.

Let's review some frequently asked questions. Are there diets that are dangerous, and how do I know? If it sounds too good to be true, it probably is.

Should children go on weight reduction diets? Yes, given the magnitude of obesity, we put children and their parents on calorie-controlled plans.

What about fasting and colon cleaning for weight reduction? These are ineffective strategies for weight control. ■

Suggested Reading

Mahan and Stump, *Krause's Food, Nutrition, and Diet Therapy*, chap. 23.

McArdle, Katch, and Katch, *Exercise Physiology*, chap. 30.

Questions to Consider

1. Which of the dietary approaches mentioned seems to be the best fit for you and members of your family?

2. If different dietary approaches are best for various members of a family, how can the main food planner and buyer manage?

Dietary Approaches to Weight Management
Lecture 23—Transcript

Welcome back. In this lecture, we're going to look at appropriate weight management strategies. I'm going to say probably most of us know someone who's been on a weight reduction diet. I had a young lady come into my office and here was her dietary strategy. To lose weight, she wasn't going to eat anything until two o'clock. After two o'clock, she was going to eat anything she wanted. That was the way that she approached weight management. Sound approach? I'm going to argue no.

In this lecture, we're going to take a look at individuals who are successful losers, using data from the National Weight Control Registry. We're also going to critique and explain some of the popular diets that are out there today, so you can become a better consumer and better informed. How do you become the biggest loser? How do you do that? Well, the National Weight Control Registry, and I would encourage everyone to go to that website and take a look at it, gives us information on what successful losers do.

First and foremost, they eat breakfast, and they eat breakfast seven out of seven days. They weigh themselves at least once a week. Why does that work? It's accountability. If I'm going to manage my calories and increase my exercise, I also have to make sure that I'm checking in and being accountable. They exercise. People on the National Weight Control Registry exercise approximately an hour, yes, an hour every day. So what that means is that they're finding the time to prioritize their health. They reduce the amount of television time to less than 10 hours per week. They do restrict calories and oftentimes just follow a low-fat diet.

The two major scientists behind this initiative are James Hill and Rena Wing. Now, again, I'm going to suggest to you check into that website. The people in the National Weight Control Registry, some of the people lose weight quickly, some of them lose it slowly, but in reality, this is a great way to say, what are the people doing who are getting this right and keeping it off? So in this National Weight Control Registry, they've been following these individuals, and these are individuals who have lost weight and kept it off. It's not just people who lose; it's successful losers.

If you want to, again, tackle this strategy of weight management, how are you going to do that? We've got a variety of different ways that you can approach it and, again, we're going to approach it with some scientific rigor. Now, you can get self-help books and manuals. You can go to the bookstore and find every book on diet that you'd ever want to, but I'm going to suggest to you critique these books like a scientist. If the pattern is unbalanced, if they're telling you to avoid major food groups, that's going to be a red flag to you that, you know what, maybe this isn't scientifically based. If it claims breakthroughs or, more importantly, says "I've got a quick fix for you" this is probably not the kind of diet that you want to be on. If it's irrational food instructions that, you know, you have to combine your foods or you can't eat this food with that food, keep in mind your gut is a very sophisticated organ, and you can really digest most food combinations. The promise of a cure for some diseases associated with weight loss, so if it says this is the diabetes cure or the cholesterol cure, you've got to start thinking to yourself maybe there's some hype associated with that.

My favorite one is this food combining theory. There are books out there now that say don't eat carbohydrate and protein together because when it gets in your gut, it putrefies and becomes rancid, and that your body can't process carbohydrates and proteins together. Well, if you think about the lecture on digestion, your body is an amazing food processing organ. Think about this—if your body couldn't digest carbohydrate and protein together, all of us, the whole entire country would be thin, so that's obviously not scientifically supported.

Some people believe that they do better with meal replacements, and what are meal replacements? Things like Slim-Fast, the drinks that come in a can. Well, they are absolutely convenient. You could bring a whole six pack into your office for a week, a little bit more than a week, so they're unbelievably convenient. The challenge with these meal replacements is, are you actually learning long-term eating strategy without the reliance on a special product? For you, if you think, "you know what? I really want to save most of my calories for the evening meal and I can get by with just a can at lunch. I really like that." I'm going to suggest this might be a good approach for you. If you actually look in the scientific literature, there is science to support the effectiveness of these meal replacement drinks.

What about self-help groups? Could you go to Overeaters Anonymous? That's generally going to suggest that food is an addiction, and for some of us it might be, so that might be a place to look. Many churches now have faith-based groups, and again, the whole idea behind it is that you have a commonality with the people that you're in this group with, and that might be a strategy to check into a church in your neighborhood, again, if you're part of that faith. The key with both OA and the faith-based groups is they provide peer support. You're in it together. It's camaraderie. It's also accountability, isn't it? If I have to go and visit with people that are, again, on a successful weight management strategy, it may provide me a little bit more motivation.

You can go to a private counselor. You can go to physicians, a psychotherapist, but I'm going to stop short of telling you to go to a nutritionist, and the reason is in the United States at this time, "nutritionist" is not a legally protected title. If you are interested in food, if you're interested in nutrition, by definition, you can call yourself a nutritionist. So what you want to look for in terms of self-help is you really want to look for a registered dietician. A registered dietician has the academic training and the clinical experience to help you navigate the waters of weight management.

You also want to have a team approach. If you're going to go to a private counselor and invest that time and money, you want someone who's going to really help you to overcome the barriers and provide an individual weight management program for you. Now, what about commercial programs?

There's Jenny Craig, there's Nutrisystem, and they provide some counseling, not done by a dietician or a physician, but by their counselors, and they provide some support and sell some prepackaged foods. If you really need to have the food delivered to your home or you pick up your food and you don't want to cook, this might be a great solution for you. Sometimes some of these programs will promote very-low-calorie diets, and they can be medically supervised or not, and they're generally liquid. You have little to no food choice. It's typically really only used as a last resort, so I don't know that I would recommend this as a first step, but it may be a step along this path. It's thought that in individuals who are really having a difficult time breaking that overeating cycle, this puts the brakes on it because you have no choice of food. It's provided for you. Again, it's usually liquid and very low calorie. The programs with the best results that provide these very-low-calorie diets are those with an interdisciplinary focus, more than one health-care provider.

What about the popular diet strategies? You've looked at self-help, you've looked at maybe a weight reduction book and you're thinking, okay, I think I'm going to start out with a popular diet. I think I'm going to do that. Well, probably the most popular, and I'm going to say probably most controversial diet over the last 30 years, and yes, Atkins keeps coming over and over and over again in different forms, is the Atkins diet. What is it? It is a low carbohydrate, ketogenic diet that says you can eat whatever you want as long as it's just from protein-containing foods. So what does "ketogenic" mean? Ketogenic means that you're burning fat faster than you can get rid of the waste products, and the waste products have rapid fat metabolism, these are ketones. Any diet that's ketogenic or supports you becoming ketotic is, again, going to be a low-carbohydrate diet. Advocates of this diet suggest the restriction of carbohydrate to 20 grams a day or less. So what does that mean in terms of practicality? A slice of bread has 15 grams of carbohydrate and a half a cup of vegetables has 5. That would be your only carbohydrate on that diet. That's it, so 20 grams is not a whole lot of carbohydrate.

What happens is that the body is now forced to come up with a different way of getting its own energy and, again, it produces ketone bodies. In theory, ketones that are lost in your urine represent unused energy. Not all the fat is going to be metabolized into usable energy, and the ketones are going to be the waste product of that. So there's some energy associated with ketones. So theoretically, it gives the Atkins devotees the idea that you can eat whatever you want, again, as long as it's going to be only protein-containing foods. The success of these diets lies in the fact that when most people decrease the amount of carbohydrate, they end up decreasing their total calorie intake. You might be a carnivore. You might really like meat, but if that's all you could eat, it may not sound so delicious. So instead of a steak and baked potato, it's steak. Instead of a grilled cheese sandwich, it's cheese. The food choices are somewhat boring, and human beings actually experience what is known as "taste fatigue." You get tired of eating the same food over and over again, and it actually becomes less delicious.

The initial weight loss on this diet is as the body is trying to clear those ketones, it has to do it with fluid. The initial weight losses on this diet are largely dehydration. I will tell you, for many individuals, that's somewhat motivating. I had a woman who was my height and 400 pounds, lost 25 pounds in the first week on this diet. Did she lose 25 pounds of body fat? No. Did she lose 25 pounds of weight? Yes, but a lot of that was fluid. Keep in mind with water loss, it reduces your scale weight, but doesn't necessarily reduce your body fat.

Low-carbohydrate diets can also cause a significant reduction in lean mass. You remember that lean mass, muscle mass, can be a source of carbohydrate. Remember what happens is that the lean mass, in the absence of carbohydrate, is sent to the liver and some of that protein can be turned into carbohydrate in order to maintain your blood sugar. Protein is a very expensive source of carbohydrate. The loss of this lean mass ends up reducing your basal metabolic rate, and that is a very undesirable effect for individuals that are looking for long-term weight loss. Remember, the more muscle mass you have, the bigger your metabolic engine. So this big metabolic engine wastes fuel. You want as much muscle mass as you can, and a low-carbohydrate diet isn't going to do that.

The Atkins diet remains credible in some eyes because you can actually see some improvement in health. How can I get some improvement in health? Remember, if you lose weight, even 5% to 10% of your body weight, you can have improvement in some of your risk factors. Certainly, some of the measures of heart disease are also going to be impacted by the Atkins diet. Some of the science will suggest that individuals that are on a low-carbohydrate diet, the Atkins diet, can actually have improvement in their triglycerides and their other lipids. So the challenge is going to be you can see an improvement in not only blood lipid profiles, but blood sugar profiles. So again, you can go to the literature and the literature will suggest individuals who stay on an Atkins diet can have improvement in their overall health.

There are medical versions of Atkins, so I'm always amazed when my colleagues say we should never recommend Atkins because in the hospital we do have something called a "protein sparing modified fast," a medical Atkins. You really have to think about long-term health, and the Atkins diet needs more long-term research on overall health risks. We know that individuals that eat all of this protein have an increased uric acid level, and remember uric acid contributes to the development of gout. It may increase the development of kidney stones because now my body has to get rid of all the extra acid. Ketones are acidic bodies. It can result in cardiac arrhythmias because it significantly alters the amount of sodium and potassium in your blood. So many people will say when they're on the Atkins diet they can feel their heart skip a beat. Again, it can cause this acidosis, which can cause damage to tissues and organs.

It may make preexisting kidney problems worse because protein waste products can only be metabolized through the kidney. So the more excess protein that I take in, I'm increasing the workload on the kidney. The other side effects are it significantly depletes the little bit of carbohydrate that you store as glycogen in your muscles and liver, and it can make you unbelievably tired. People that are on low-carbohydrate diets really have exercise intolerance. They can't go out and exercise at the same rate.

Because there is no low-fat dairy on this diet, it reduces calcium balance and can increase your risk of bone loss. We know, maybe it's intended and unintended, it results in dehydration. To me as a dietician, one of the things that's most concerning to me is the absence of fruits and vegetables. Fruits and vegetables are that natural anti-inflammatory, and keep in mind heart disease, cancer, and most chronic illnesses have inflammation as part of their pathophysiology. I've got no buffer. I have nothing that's going to prevent me from having an inflammatory response.

What about other ways? If we step outside of Atkins, again, very-low-calorie diets and very-low-carbohydrate diets certainly can be under strict medical supervision. When would you use something like that? When would you use a very-low-calorie diet, something that's under 1000 calories a day? In individuals that have severe clinical obesity, a BMI of at least greater than 35, may be a candidate for one of these programs. The advocates of these programs will suggest you're going to limit your daily calorie intake to between 400 and 800 calories. It's going to be mostly high quality protein-containing foods, and these diets actually came out maybe 30 years ago. The early versions of these were in a mystery liquid form that, unbeknownst to the consumer, the protein that was in these foods was ground up animal hooves, horns, pigskin mixed with some enzymes and tenderizers to predigest it. I don't know about you, but that doesn't sound terribly delicious to me.

These liquids were largely collagen-based and didn't contain all the essential amino acids. What does that mean? If you reflect back to the protein lecture, if I don't have all the essential amino acids in the right amount, protein synthesis stops. So individuals that were on these earlier diets had abnormalities in their EKG. They had copper deficiencies. They had an increased heart rate. But now we have much better versions, much more improved versions, and probably the most popular one is Medifast.

Do we have some common sense approaches? If we don't want to do the dieting extreme, what else can we do? Weight Watchers is probably one of the most successful commercial programs out there, and for good reason. It contains all the components of a successful diet. It's calorie managed, it promotes recipe development, it promotes accountability, it's calorie restriction, accountability, and support. Again, those are the hallmarks of successful programs. You can get recipes and tips during weigh-ins, and you can certainly now do Weight Watchers online.

Another diet approach that I really like is the South Beach diet. It's written by a cardiologist, so that's going to amp it up a little bit, and it's low glycemic. Remember, low-glycemic-index diets are ones that the carbohydrate is processed slowly. It blunts that insulin response. For individuals who tend to accumulate their weight in their gut, they tend to have that belly fat, a low-glycemic-index diet might be a good strategy. There's also a cookbook associated with it, and some meal plans. I've actually cooked foods from the cookbook and they're absolutely delicious.

When you're trying to, as a consumer, think, what's the newest and latest, greatest diet book that's out there? How can someone critique this for me? You can check the great diet book review on the website of the American

Dietetic Association. American Dietetic Association's website is at www. eatright.org, and every year, they're going to review the latest and greatest diet book and give you a critique. Keep in mind all diets are going to work if you follow them.

We've got to come up with this, what about exercise again? Although exercise is not a popular diet, it's not going to be Weight Watchers, it's not going to be South Beach, the amount of calories that you actually burn in exercise is relatively low. If that's your primary weight loss strategy, I think you're going to be disappointed. Remember, you burn about 100 calories per mile of walking, so let's do the math. I eat a 900-calorie slice of cheesecake and yes, if you get cheesecake in a restaurant, it can be 900 calories. I'm going to suggest you serve that to a family of four. That's not a singular portion. If you do the math, you've got to walk 9 miles. Well, I don't know about you, I'm not going to walk nine miles if I eat a 900-calorie slice of cheesecake, and most people out-eat their exercise.

In order to prevent weigh regain after weight loss, exercise is absolutely key. Remember the National Weight Control Registry? Again, exercise may also aid in the loss of visceral or belly fat, and interval training, where you walk and then maybe job for 30 seconds, and walk and jog may be the most desirable form. Well is there anything else? If I've tried this, I've tried commercial products, I've tried a lot of other things, what about over-the-counter drugs and dietary supplements? Remember, the dieting industry has the most fraud associated with it, so again, if you're putting on your detective hat, you've got to think, okay, could there be fraud in these over-the-counter drugs and dietary supplements? Well, many of the weight loss supplements contain caffeine in some way, shape, or form. You might not recognize it. Sources of caffeine include guarana, they include cola nut, they include yerba maté—these are words that don't roll off the tongue of most Americans. Caffeine is a stimulant and a diuretic in large amounts, so that might be a strategy for weight control. I don't know about you, but if I consumed a whole lot of caffeine, it might be a little nauseating to me, and that would also blunt my appetite.

Benzocaine is actually added to a lot of the weight loss products, and I love this strategy. Benzocaine is a topical numbing agent. The strategy is, I'm going to numb your tongue and hopefully reduce the way the food tastes and discourage eating. Well, I liken that to going and having dental work at the dentist, and they inject you with a numbing agent, and you end up biting your tongue, so maybe that would work, I don't know.

There are fiber pills out there, and we do know that fiber helps in its natural form in fruits and vegetables and whole grains. That does promote fullness. A fiber pill is going to be encapsulated fiber, and I'm going to have to drink a lot of water in order to get that gut expansion, and I've seen some really disastrous consequences of people taking fiber pills with inadequate water. Now, certainly, the theory behind this is if I fill up your belly enough, you're going to have less of an appetite. Some of that's true, but again, this combination where I might be getting caffeine, benzocaine, and fiber all in one pill can actually lead to some dehydration. And, again, remember, the scale can move, but if it's dehydration, I haven't lost body fat.

Very few studies have evaluated any of these over-the-counter products for weight loss, and there's little evidence to promote their use. Is there anything else? Yeah, there is.

There was a product on the market, and I'm going to tell you it's coming back, called "ephedra." In 2004, the FDA, the Food and Drug Administration, actually banned the use of ephedra. Ephedra does show short-term weight loss, so is it an effective supplement? Absolutely, but it's absolutely dangerous to people with hypertension, heart disease, or diabetes, so I think the challenge is that ephedra was removed from the market in 2004. And it's now creeping back in. And certainly, the Internet is going to be a place where a lot of people are going to end up getting ephedra. You can get a lot of things on the Internet that you really shouldn't be able to get, and ephedra's a great example.

What about anti-obesity drugs? Do we have anything that we can actually use? Yes, we do. There are two that are approved by the FDA. One is called "Meridia," and the generic name for that is "sibutramine," and Xenical, or orlistat, are approved for long-term treatment. Meridia is an appetite suppressant that actually affects the chemicals in the brain. But it will increase blood pressure, so if you're hypertensive, if you have high blood pressure, Meridia might not be for you. It increases blood pressure and increases heart rate, and again, some public interest groups have asked the government to take it off the market. The problem is I can get anything on the Internet. I can get anything on the Internet, and that's going to become important in just a minute.

Xenical actually interferes with pancreatic lipase, and pancreatic lipase—remember, "ase" is an enzyme—digests fat, and it interferes with fat digestion and can reduce the absorption of fat by up to 30%. Well, anytime I malabsorb fat, I'm going to also lose those fat-soluble vitamins. In 2002, there was some research suggesting it improved weight loss by 2% to 3%. You can now get Xenical or orlistat in an over-the-counter version called "alli," and again, alli, orlistat, xenical all have to be consumed with a low-fat diet. So the biggest problem with alli is it causes fat malabsorption, and the side effects can be significant and really difficult to manage. Oily diarrhea comes to mind. It's causing fat malabsorption. If I decide I'm going to take alli and go out and eat a cheese pizza, I'm going to be stuck in my house because the diarrhea becomes uncontrollable.

The FDA always suggests with any of these anti-obesity drugs, you've got to do them in concert with a low-calorie diet. Now, that Internet is going to come up over and over again. You can actually buy amphetamines over the Internet. You can Meridia over the Internet without a physician's prescription. I've tried to do that multiple times, and I can buy anything. Again, I think the real challenge is you can buy addictive drugs. Your children or grandchildren can buy addictive drugs, i.e. amphetamines, off the Internet and you've got to be really very vigilant about that. Again, amphetamines are an addictive drug.

The benefits of drug therapy over behavioral modification interventions are modest at best, so most people can't live on amphetamines. Yes, you'll lose weight, but most people can't live on them. What's our last stop on this road? We've looked at popular diets; we've looked at ketogenic diets, behavioral support, Weight Watchers. The last resort is going to be surgery, and it can be effective in individuals who have what is called "morbid obesity," a BMI of greater than 40. It really should be a last effort after all legitimate efforts have been tried.

I'm going to tell you there have been times where I'll say, there is no other solution. Remember my biggest man? The biggest man was 1065 pounds. In him, gastric surgery is lifesaving. Now, there's gastric banding, and what gastric banding does is reduces the size of the stomach by creating a smaller upper stomach. So that's going to actually be advantageous. You see this with gastric banding and gastric bypass. If I reduce the stomach size, I can reduce food intake. If I have gastric bypass, I can actually bypass some of that small intestine. Remember that most of the digestion and absorption in your whole GI tract occurs in the small intestine, so if I bypass the small intestine by surgical rerouting, I will end up with not only a smaller intake, small stomach, but I'm also going to malabsorb, or lose some of those calories when I have a bowel movement, because I've bypassed some of the intestine.

What are the results with gastric bypass or gastric banding? Patients lose substantially more weight in the initial phases than those just using exercise and a proper diet. However, the weight loss tends to plateau between a year and a half and two years, but most patients can maintain about 50% of that initial body weight loss after five years. However, I've actually had a patient who now is on her third gastric bypass. She figured out ways of just getting in very-high-calorie liquid foods, milkshakes, ice cream, things such as that. So the long-term effectiveness of this program depends on how people manage their eating. You've got to exercise, you've got to stay away from those really calorie-dense foods, the milkshakes, the ice creams, and again, there are no long-term studies on bariatric surgery and pregnancy, for example.

I'm going to suggest to you that there are other ways that people try and reshape their body. Liposuction actually just sucks out body fat. That's not effective as a long-term solution. In fact, it's generally not recommended for individuals who really are having a hard time with this weight cycling—their weight's going up and down—because you can get a really cosmetically poor effect if I suck out fat and then I replace it with more. It's not effective as a long-term treatment. The risks include blood clots, perforation injuries, skin and nerve damage, and, again, unfavorable drug reactions for some of the medications that are used.

What does work? Decrease your energy intake by 500 to 1000 calories below daily expenditure. Moderately restricting food intake is a plan because if I severely restrict it, I'm not going to be able to stay with that long enough. If I moderately restrict my food intake, I'm going to have a greater fat loss than with a drastic energy restriction. People who create large daily deficits tend to lose weight more rapidly, but they also regain it, and that's what we want to avoid doing.

Keep tabs on your habits and become involved in other activities other than eating, especially something with fitness. Long-term success depends on maintaining the lifestyle changes that helped you to lose weight originally. For the best effect, weight management plans must be individualized, so I think that's a real key point. If you've tried everything, you may want to go and think, "I need to have something that's going to fit me and it's going to fit my lifestyle."

Now we're going to talk about those frequently asked questions, the kinds of things that I see in my clinical practice all the time. Are there diets that are dangerous, and how do I know? Again, be a detective. If it sounds too good to be true, if this diet approach is promising you the sun, the stars, and the moon, you've got to think, "Okay, first of all, that isn't going to work, and second of all, it has the potential to be dangerous if it's really restricting a significant amount of food."

Here's a really touchy subject. Should children go on weight reduction diets? I have to tell you, years ago, I would have said no. I would have said, "absolutely not. Let them grow into their weight." What I see now, though, is girls and, again, my youngest girl with type 2 diabetes at Texas Children's is four. She's 120 pounds. She's going to have to be an adult before she grows into that weight, and so in someone like that, I would suggest, yeah, they have to go on a weight reduction diet. The science of children and weight management is just so concerning because children that are obese in elementary school are bullied. They're teased. They're less likely to go to prom or dances. They're less likely to be invited to social interactions. And so I think the challenge is, what do we do for individuals like that? And I've now reversed my philosophy, given the magnitude of obesity that I see, and now we'll put children on calorie-controlled plans, and probably more importantly, I put their parents on calorie-controlled plans.

What about fasting and colon cleaning for weight reduction? Absolutely not. If you're fasting for religious reasons, I support that. But to fast for weight control or to do a colon cleanse, colon cleanses are just going to dehydrate you because they're cleaning out your large intestine, and where is food absorbed? Small intestine. It's an ineffective strategy for weight control. I can change the scale weight, but I can't change the body weight. Fasting, as we know, for weight control only is going to chew up functional lean mass, and that's really what we want to avoid.

The common sense things—eat less, exercise more, be vigilant—always rule the day. Thank you very much.

Nutrition and Cancer Prevention
Lecture 24

Prostate cancer is the leading form in men, and breast cancer is the leading form in women. Poor diet is estimated to account for 30%–35% of cancer cases.

Currently, cancer is the second leading cause of death in the United States. We explore the dietary strategies and lifestyle modifications needed to reduce cancer risk and touch on modifying these recommendations if the diagnosis of cancer has been made.

Cancer is cells gone wild. Our cells are constantly being exposed to DNA-damaging events such as sun exposure, tobacco, environmental chemicals, and alcohol. Damaged cells can have 2 specific fates: apoptosis or cell multiplication. When this aberrant cell growth develops its own blood supply, it is cancer. Eliminating tobacco, alcohol, and sun exposure can help prevent cancer.

Cancer is cells gone wild.

Food and nutrition can either act as a cancer cell promoter or killer. Diet and weight management can aid in the prevention of cancer. A plant-based diet might aid in cancer prevention as well. Mortality rates from both heart disease and cancer increase in tandem with red meat consumption. Reduce meat consumption and avoid grilling, since charred meat can increase the risk of cancer. Eat more whole grains. Regarding cancer prevention, the best approach is no alcohol. Avoid cured meats. Nitrosamines are cancer-causing compounds that are formed when meats are cured.

There are anticancer compounds in fruits and vegetables. When you are organizing your plant-based meals, color and variety of colors matter. Indoles, found in white and green cruciferous vegetables, downregulate the production of one of the stages of cell division in the cancer process. Indoles can also alter the effects of estrogen and promote cancer cell apoptosis. Lycopene is the red pigment in tomatoes, pink grapefruit, and watermelon and has multiple roles in the prevention of cancer.

83

For the color gold, try turmeric: It has curcurmin, which is thought to induce cell apoptosis. However, it may reduce the effectiveness of chemotherapy. Yellow and orange produce, such as carrots, corn, and cantaloupe, have carotenoids, which were found to decrease the risk of breast cancer in postmenopausal women.

For blues, purples, and additional reds, try blueberries, raspberries, and strawberries. These contain anthocyanins, which can repair the DNA damage that is the first step of cancer development. Green tea is rich in polyphenolic compounds, most notably catechins, which can induce apoptosis.

The double-edged sword here is soy. Whole soy may be protective against the development of breast cancer, but those who have breast cancer should probably avoid soy isoflavones.

Vitamins may play a role in the prevention of cancer. Folic acid is needed for DNA synthesis and may help in the prevention of pancreatic and colon cancer. Low levels of folic acid have been linked with breast cancer. Vitamin D from sunlight or from supplements may be effective in the prevention of breast cancer. However, data from the Women's Health Initiative showed no

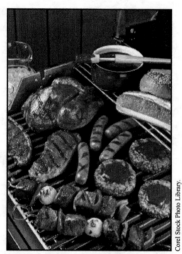

Grilling, and particularly marinating, can increase the charring of meat, which can increase the risk of cancer.

such effects. The American Cancer Society study suggested that those who take vitamin E for 10 years may reduce the risk of bladder cancer; however, the SELECT study demonstrated that taking vitamin E and selenium together was not an effective strategy for the prevention of prostate cancer.

Here are our take-home points: Control your weight, your life, and your food. Choose plant-based foods and beverages from the colors of the rainbow.

Let's review some frequently asked questions. What about nutritional needs during and after chemotherapy and radiation treatments for cancer? Your needs depend on the type of cancer and treatment—always consult your doctor or dietician.

Does coffee have any cancer-fighting properties? Coffee consumption may reduce the risk of liver cancer, but it may be associated with an increased risk of lung cancer.

Can I use a supplement for vitamin D if I am following the American Cancer Society's recommendation to avoid exposure to the sun? Yes. ■

Suggested Reading

Brown, J., *Nutrition Now*, unit 23.

Duyff, *American Dietetic Association Complete Food and Nutrition Guide*, chap. 22.

Questions to Consider

1. What nutrition and lifestyle steps can you take to prevent cancer?

2. Even if you take those steps toward cancer prevention, why is it still important to have regular checkups and testing?

Nutrition and Cancer Prevention
Lecture 24—Transcript

Greetings, and welcome back. I'm going to start out today with a little different story. I'm going to give you my personal experience with cancer. It was January, 2004, and I was in my office. I had just visited my OB/GYN in December. When I got the call, "Roberta, you have breast cancer," I will tell you it took my breath away. First, I started thinking, "oh my goodness, I'm a mother. I'd love to be a grandmother. I'd love to see my children get married." All the thoughts that all of us are going to have when we're diagnosed with a potentially life-threatening disease. When I got myself together, I went and told my boss, and I immediately left and used all my connections and got in at MD Anderson.

But somewhere in that process, I started thinking, why me? I exercise. I eat well. Why me? And so after the "why me?" was over, and the pity party stopped, I thought, I have the ability to tackle this with good nutrition, with exercise, and with my great medical team. And so I'm happy to say that I am a cancer survivor, but I will say for myself and maybe many of you all, I will say this was a life-changing event. I will never look at a patient again the same way because once those words, "you have cancer" hit me, I stopped in my tracks and I wasn't really able to hear the rest of the conversation. So it was a personal, terrifying journey, but one that I actually will say made me a better clinician in the long run.

Currently, cancer is the second leading cause of death in the United States, and the most feared diagnosis. Although heart disease is the number one killer of Americans, the diagnosis of cancer for me, and many Americans, is terrifying. In men, prostate cancer is the leading form of cancer, and for women, it's breast cancer. Certainly, we have lots of public health campaigns to alert women to the dangers of breast cancer and the need for screening. However, we don't have the same vigilance when it comes to prostate cancer in men. Historically, prostate cancer is more common in men than breast cancer has been in women. However, of the cancers diagnosed in the year 2008, 25% of the new cancers in men were prostate, and 26% were breast cancer in women. So clearly, we have some work to do in the prevention of cancer.

Poor diet is estimated to account for 30% to 35% of the cancers, and therefore we can do something to modify our risk. But please keep in mind, just like me, modification of risk does not preclude the need for early detection and diagnosis. I was the one that found my breast cancer. It did not appear on a mammogram. I found it through a regular breast exam. So again, please remember that although you might do everything possible in terms of diet and exercise, please make sure that you keep up with diagnostic testing. Additionally, outside of diet, there are other lifestyle risk factors, such as tobacco use, alcohol consumption, and lack of exercise that can increase the overall risk of almost all cancers.

What's the focus of this lecture? This lecture is going to explore the dietary strategies and lifestyle modifications needed to reduce cancer risk. And we're also going to touch on modifying these recommendations if the diagnosis of cancer has been made. So do you do something differently? But to understand this, we have to understand the process of cancer development, and I think what this will do is reinforce to you that all of us need to have regular health exams and regular screening.

What is cancer? Simply stated, cancer is cells gone wild, cells that are misbehaving and not doing what they're supposed to do. All of us, and all of our cells, are constantly being exposed to DNA-damaging events, so somewhere in our environment, we all have damage to our DNA. And what are these kinds of damaging events? Well, certainly, sun exposure. If you're out in the sun, you can damage skin cells. You can damage the DNA in those cells and, again, increase your risk of cancer. Tobacco in all forms, and I had a young man in my class at Rice and he was a baseball player. He would come to class chewing tobacco. So one day after class, I said, "I've love to take you on a field trip." So we took a field trip to MD Anderson and went to the oral cancer section. He saw firsthand what happens when you chew tobacco, the damage that can be done to your oral cavity, a tongue resection. And I will tell you that was probably an "Aha" moment for him, that maybe, even though most baseball players may do this, this might not be what's best for him.

Certainly, environmental chemicals. For me, I worked in a nutrition lab in graduate school and I was exposed to a lot of environmental chemicals.

Alcohol can be this DNA-damaging event. When we cluster all of these together, these events are known as "initiation." This is the entrance into cancer, and again, all of us can't look into our historical crystal ball and say what our initiating event was, but chances are we've all had one. Well, under genetic control and complex cell machinery, the damaged cells can have either of two specific fates. It can go in two different directions.

It can go to cell death. The cell line can die off and this is known as "apoptosis." The normal cell mechanisms can't repair the cell and it dies. Or it can also progress, this damaged cell can progress and the cell can multiply. This is where we have a little bit of a concern because again, we can't look into our cell machinery and say, "which fate did my damaged cell have?" So it can either go to apoptosis or it can progress and the cell can multiply. The development of a blood supply to this aberrant cell growth is what we call cancer. So again, we've all had these initiating events. Hopefully, our cell machinery is great and that cell line dies off, but if the cell line goes wild and develops its own blood supply, that's known as cancer.

Tumors appear to be made of many different types of cells, including precancerous stem cells, and this was first discovered in leukemia. These stem cells have the characteristics of both abnormal and normal cells. Some science suggests that these stem cells that are kind of hiding and lurking in the background, with characteristics of both abnormal and normal cells, are one of the reasons why cancer can return. Okay, let's get to the nuts and bolts.

What about cancer prevention? Well, just like my Rice baseball player, elimination of tobacco in all forms. No form of tobacco is safe. Keep in mind, tobacco can be an initiating event. This is particularly deadly when you combine it with alcohol. Both tobacco and alcohol are thought to initiate and promote cancer development, so you get a deadly two-for-the-price-of-one here. Not only do they cause cell damage, but they also actually promote cancer development.

Additionally, the American Cancer Society suggests that 1 million skin cancers could be prevented by eliminating sun exposure. Now, in our lecture on vitamin D, again, this is a double-edged sword because we know that the sun is a great source of vitamin D. So by eliminating sun exposure, you can also eliminate one of your major sources of vitamin D. Sunscreen can be very effective for preventing skin cancer, but it must be applied in an appropriate way, with the higher the SPF rating, in general, the better. Exposure to UV light in tanning salons can be just as dangerous as exposure to the sun itself, so for those of you who want that overall glow, maybe you use a topical, fake suntan and get it that way, rather than risking going to a tanning salon.

Some of the more exciting things in terms of cancer development is that now we know that certain viruses have been implicated in cervical cancer, and possibly some other cancers as well. The new Gardasil vaccine can be given to prevent certain forms, but not all forms, of cervical cancer caused by the HPV virus.

What about food and healthy lifestyles? The current thinking is that food and nutrition can either act as a cancer cell promoter—it can force that cell line into the development of cancer—or a cancer cell killer—it can promote apoptosis. According to the American Cancer Society, diet and weight management can aid in the prevention of cancer. Think about it this way. If you're struggling with weight management and you're struggling with exercise, you might want to think about this as your deposit in the cancer prevention bank. You really want to look at that in a positive way and maybe it might change the way that you look at some of your favorite, although not healthy, foods.

Exercise most days of the week, and in this case, there appears to be a dose-related response. What does that mean? It means 30 minutes is good, but an hour would be better. Human bodies are designed to move, and apparently, in this case, what is happening is that in individuals who do not exercise, they become resistant to insulin, so they make more insulin. Remember our lecture on pre-diabetes and metabolic syndrome? Insulin is an anabolic hormone. Anabolic means building. And what you're doing is promoting cancer development when you don't exercise. You are increasing insulin resistance. Your body makes more insulin. Insulin is an anabolic hormone that promotes cancer development. So exercise, again, is part of that ticket to good health.

Let's make some simple recommendations because simple recommendations matter. How about thinking of a plant-based diet? Again, over and over, this comes up in normal nutrition and disease prevention. A plant-based diet means the more of your plate that is occupied by vegetables, the better. One way that you might want to think about this is thinking about having a meatless Monday, where your main dish on Monday night might be vegetarian. Now, by vegetarian, I'm talking about beans and tofu, and not necessarily just cheese or other high-fat foods. This term "meatless Monday" was first coined by a group of nutrition professionals at Johns Hopkins, and I use this a lot in my clinical practice. Can I get you to eat vegetarian one night per week? Additionally, what I'm doing is helping people to choose different foods that maybe they haven't tried before. So maybe it's a veggie burger that you have. That might be a way of looking at it, with a big plate of three-bean salad to go along with it.

A recent study in the Archives of Internal Medicine, which included more than a half-million subjects, so this should make you pause a second because keep in mind, this is a large number of people, suggested that those who consume the highest amount of red meat have a higher mortality rate. This study is known as the "NIH-AARP Diet and Health Study." Mortality rates from both heart disease and cancer were increased with increasing red meat consumption. So what are some big recommendations from this study? Reduce the meat and avoid grilling. Grilling, and particularly marinating, can increase the charring of that grilled meat. But it appears that beer and wine-based marinades might actually reduce the risk, and the science is still emerging on this.

It is the charred meat that can increase the risk of cancer. The increase in high temperatures with high-protein foods increases the production of what are known as "heterocyclic amines." They are the charred byproducts of grilling. Now, say for example, you're invited over to somebody's house. They're not really great with their grilling skills and you've got everything that is significantly blackened. Trim off as much of that as you can. Trim off the blackened piece and maybe flavor it up with a little bit more barbeque sauce, but trim of the burned portion and reduce the consumption of heterocyclic amines.

Once again, eating more whole grains matters in terms of cancer prevention. What's the etiology or what's the mechanism behind this? Well, this could easily be that whole grains are going to have more fiber. Whole grains are possibly going to be, again, this wonderful compound called a "pre-biotic," food for the probiotics, and that might be it, or maybe it's an individual nutrient within the whole grains. Maybe it's magnesium here, raising its head in whole grains. Again, eating more whole grains is going to make a difference as well. So these are part of our simple recommendations.

Regarding alcohol use in cancer prevention, the best approach is no alcohol because keep in mind, alcohol, at least minimally, is going to serve as an initiating event. But if you do drink alcohol, the recommendation is to limit your intake to one drink per day for women, and two for men. Certainly, avoid cured meats. These are processed meats, such as bacon, ham, and hot dogs, and I'm going to caution you here. As individuals, try and get away from beef and pork. We now have cured turkey products. We have turkey hot dogs and everyone believes, again, because of that singular first ingredient, "oh, turkey has to be better for me." Well, the problem is it's the curing of the meat that is going to increase cancer risk as well. Nitrosamines are cancer-causing compounds that are formed when meats are cured, and these should be limited in everyone's diet. Certainly, think of things that you might have at a picnic. Are we always going to have hot dogs and cured meats, or can we come up with some other strategies?

There is more, and this is probably the good news to the story. There are magical compounds, and I really do call them "magical," in fruits and vegetables. The colors of the rainbow represent the pot of gold at the end of the fruit and vegetable and plant-based diet. I want you to think when you're organizing your plant-based meals, color and variety of colors matter. So let's explore some of those. First and foremost, we're going to take a look at a compound called "indoles." Indoles are the whites and the greens. These are also known as "cruciferous vegetables," so things like broccoli, cauliflower, cabbage, and kale. Those are all, again, the whites and the greens.

I'll tell you, when I first started my career in nutrition, we would say, "well, cauliflower is good for you, but because it doesn't have enough vitamin C, or fill in the vitamin, we really don't think you need to consume much cauliflower." It's not the vitamins in the fruits and the vegetables that are cancer preventers. Most of the vitamin studies have fallen short. It's the colors. It's the pigments. It's the words we can't pronounce that oftentimes are going to be the nutritional heroes in fruits and vegetables. What do these compounds do? What do indoles do? They downregulate or reduce the production of one of the stages of cell division in the cancer process. We also know that indoles can act as negative estrogen regulators, and alter the effects of estrogen and promote cancer cell apoptosis.

Let's think about this one for a second. Most of the breast cancer in women is estrogen receptor positive. So what that means is that you are vulnerable, as a woman, to increased risk of breast cancer, you are vulnerable to the increased amounts of estrogen. So what that means is if indoles can actually downregulate that estrogen receptor, it may reduce your risk of the most common form of breast cancer. Research also suggests that they can be invaluable in the prevention of cervical cancer, particularly in those who have what is called "precancerous cervical dysplasia." They're already in that suspicious range, and the indoles may be preventative.

Certainly, there's a potential role in the prevention of prostate cancer. So again, if we pause and think breast cancer is most common in women, prostate in men, think about if there creative ways that you can eat more broccoli and cabbage? Coleslaw would be a great example of where you could introduce some cabbage into someone's diet that may not like it.

Continuing on the colors of the rainbow, lycopene is the red pigment. I want you to think if the food is red, it rules. Things like tomatoes, pink grapefruit, and watermelon, all of those are great red foods. I've been asked if juices of these fruits and vegetables are beneficial. Certainly, the whole food is preferred, but in a pinch, juices can serve as a reasonable substitute. So let's say you're travelling and you don't have the availability of a fresh salad, but you decide you're going to grab a can of tomato juice. That would be a really great plan. It's not quite as good, but it's almost as good as the whole fruit or vegetable.

Multiple roles exist for lycopene in the prevention of cancer. It acts as an antioxidant, protecting those wonderful cell membranes. It may prevent the abnormal cell division. Large epidemiological studies show a relationship between those who have low levels of lycopene in their blood and an increased prevalence of prostate cancer, so there appears to be a relationship. However, currently, studies have not demonstrated the prevention of prostate cancer through increased consumption of lycopene, but again, the science is emerging on this topic, so stay tuned. Cooked tomato products actually have an increased amount of bioavailable lycopene, so here's an example where raw is not going to be as good as cooked. So when you're having your meatless Monday and you're trying a veggie burger, put ketchup on it. How many times have you heard a dietician say, "use a condiment to prevent cancer"? Probably not too many times.

Spice up your food with some additional color. So as we think about the colors of the rainbow, think gold. Turmeric, which is a traditional curry spice, is actually a cancer prevention powerhouse. The active compound is curcurmin, and curcurmin is again, thought to induce cell apoptosis, have that aberrant cell die rather than proliferate. It is best studied in colon cancer and leukemia, so again, maybe on your meatless Monday, you might want to try a chickpea curry, and add some turmeric to it, to have a double cancer-preventing diet.

However, as we discover with many dietary compounds, there can be some downsides to using turmeric, and here's an example. Turmeric, particularly when it's used as a supplement and not as a spice, may reduce the effectiveness of chemotherapy. So here's the pause. Sometimes compounds that are needed for the prevention of cancer actually are not a good idea during cancer treatment. This is where you need to talk to your physician, visit a registered dietician, because again, what is sometimes good for prevention may not be so good during treatment.

What about yellow and orange produce, such as carrots, and corn, and cantaloupe? In a recent study published in *The American Journal of Clinical Nutrition*, carotenoids were found to decrease the risk of breast cancer in postmenopausal women. Remember, it's the carotenoids that are the yellow orange pigments, so the carotenoids may reduce the risk of breast cancer in postmenopausal women.

What about the other colors of the rainbow? How about some blues and purples and some additional reds? Pretty simply stated, think berries. Berries such as blueberries, and again, I started out in graduate school and we were actually told, "don't waste your calories on blueberries because there really is no nutrition in blueberries." And now they have ramped up on the scale, again, not because of their vitamin content, but because of a compound called anthocyanins. Anthocyanins in blueberries, raspberries, and strawberries actually contain wonderful phytochemicals that can repair the DNA damage. So again, you've had this initiating event. You're trying to salvage that cell and to the rescue come the berries. Remember that the damage to DNA cells is the first step of cancer development. So these berries have the potential to stop cancer in its tracks.

What about green tea? Anybody up for green tea? Tea, outside of water, is the most popular beverage in the world. It is brewed from the leaves of the *Camellia sinensis* plant. Tea is rich in polyphenolic compounds, most notably catechins and EGCG. You might see EGCG added to diet products because there's also a thought that this rich polyphenolic compound, EGCG, may actually stimulate your metabolic rate. Although that might be true, it's a slight increase in your metabolic rate, and doesn't give you license to go out and eat that 900-calorie slice of cheesecake. These compounds in tea can prevent the development of dangerous cell lines by, again, inducing apoptosis.

The double-edged sword here is soy. It contains a group of compounds known as "isoflavones," and these compounds may have estrogen-like effects. But here is, again, what the American consumer has done. In most of our dietary backgrounds, we did not grow up eating soy, tofus, miso, tempeh, and so we don't necessarily have a taste for soy. What we've done is take a wonderful food like whole soy and try to dissect out the active ingredients. And now what we have in a lot of energy bars and nutrition bars are a group of compounds called "soy isoflavones."

The real dilemma is whole soy may be protective against the development of breast cancer, but now we have a little bit of concern for those who may actually have breast cancer. The compounds that are thought to be active in soy are called "genistein," "daidzein," and "glycitein." Again, all these words that we cannot pronounce. Genistein has been shown to slow cell cancer growth in, again, this aberrant cell line. I think the challenge, however, is that you have to look at this and think, okay, where did it show cell growth or the slowing of cell growth? It's generally in the test tube. One of the concerns is, is it the whole soy that we should be looking at? Again, many breast cancers are estrogen-positive, which means you probably shouldn't be using these soy isoflavones.

Certainly, however, we may want to reduce the risk of prostate cancer, so think about this for a second. If a good percentage of breast cancer is estrogen-positive, that means many prostate cancers are testosterone fueled. So soy in the prevention of prostate cancer may work from a different mechanism. How does that work? Again, it's going to compete with testosterone. Genistein, again, one of these wonderful, active ingredients in soy, may actually interfere with one of the most popular breast cancer drugs, tamoxifen. So again, where whole soy may help prevent breast cancer, a soy protein isolate, or an isoflavone, may actually interfere with tamoxifen treatment.

What role do vitamins play? Like other food-based compounds, vitamins may play a role in the prevention of cancer. Folic acid is one. Folic acid is a B vitamin and it is needed for DNA synthesis. A major study in China has linked low levels of folic acid with breast cancer, meaning if you have a low level of folic acid in your blood, it increases the risk of breast cancer. Folic acid may also help in the prevention of pancreatic and colon cancer. Now, again, a lot of this is dependant on when you were exposed to low levels of folic acid, and that's going to be an important consideration. However, a popular chemotherapeutic agent, a drug to treat cancer, and a standard treatment for rheumatoid arthritis, methotrexate, works as a folic acid antagonist.

I want you to think about this. Why would you give a vitamin antagonist for the treatment of cancer? Well, if cancer needs folic acid to divide and replicate, if I remove folic acid from the milieu, if I remove the folic acid, i.e. methotrexate, I can actually promote cell death. The problem is your healthy cells also need folic acid, and this is one of the reasons why individuals oftentimes lose hair or have mouth ulcers as part of cancer treatment. The normal healthy cells are deprived of folic acid in an attempt to remove it from a cancer cell and stop its growth. Now, think about this for a second. If you decide you're using methotrextate for, let's say, rheumatoid arthritis, the addition of folic acid to the diet of someone using methotrexate may actually reduce the effectiveness of the drug.

Do we have other vitamin heroes in the prevention of cancer? Vitamin D from sunlight or from supplements may be effective in the prevention of breast cancer. This is supported by the fact that many women with active breast cancer were shown to be deficient in this vitamin. Keep in mind, reflect back to the vitamin lecture. One of the things that vitamin D does is it teaches cells what they should become. It helps the cell to have normal differentiation. It is the conductor of the orchestra, so it sends the cell in the direction it should be. In the absence of vitamin D, the thought it, what's going to happen here? If I don't have adequate amounts of vitamin D, this cell may not have its normal differentiation process, and it may go on to form an aberrant cell line.

However, as with folic acid, sometimes the results of studies are less than convincing. Data from the Women's Health Initiative showed no effects in terms of cancer prevention. Also, in men with aggressive prostate cancer, the higher blood levels of vitamin D are associated with an increased mortality. Recall a previous lecture on vitamin E and its effectiveness in cancer prevention. The American Cancer Society study suggested that those who take vitamin E for 10 years may reduce the risk of bladder cancer. But again, on the other hand, and this is the way clinical nutrition always is, the SELECT study demonstrated that taking vitamin E and selenium together was not an effective strategy for the prevention of prostate cancer.

Do we have any take-home points? How do we sort the nuts from the berries? First and foremost, control your weight, your life, and your food. Easy for me to say, not so easy to do. Choose plant-based foods and beverages. Think fruits and vegetables first, and think about how easy this would be. You go to a buffet and everyone tells me, oh, the buffet is the worst. I will tell you, a buffet should be the easiest place because what you do is you think, okay, I'm on my cancer prevention diet. I'm going to have at least 50% of my plate as fruits and vegetables, and then I'll fill—I call it backfilling—the rest of my plate with some of my favorite foods, but I want to make sure that I frontload my plate with lots of fruits and vegetables. Choose from the colors of the rainbow. As we've learned, multiple wonderful phytochemicals in fruits and vegetables, vitamins and minerals in fruits and vegetables, that may be linked with the prevention of cancer.

Frequently asked questions. What about nutritional needs during and after chemotherapy and radiation treatments for cancer? There are changes in nutritional needs, depending on the type of cancer and, more importantly, the type of treatment. For me personally, I did not do chemotherapy. I caught my cancer early. It was not a very aggressive form, and so I just did six weeks of radiation. In radiation, you're having significant cell damage, so making sure that you have a diet rich in fruits and vegetables to promote the healing of that damaged tissue is really pretty important, plus increasing water is important to get rid of the waste products from radiation. But when you are trying to customize—because cancer is not a homogenous term, it is very heterogeneous—there's more than one type of breast cancer, more than one type of prostate cancer. So always consult your physician or a dietician for a more customized dietary program.

Beverages. I'm asked questions all the time. I love coffee. Can you give me some justification? Does coffee have any cancer-fighting properties? Well, studies have shown that coffee consumption up to two cups a day may actually reduce the risk of liver cancer. Keep in mind, because coffee is plant-based, it's going to have phytochemicals. It's going to have wonderful polyphenolic compounds that may actually help in cancer prevention. However, another study revealed that coffee may be associated with an increased risk of lung cancer. Keep in mind some of the compounds in coffee are antioxidants, and we learned with beta-carotene, another antioxidant, that that also increases the risk of lung cancer.

How would I get vitamin D, is another popular question. I'm avoiding the sunlight. I'm following the American Cancer Society's recommendation to avoid exposure to the sun. Can I use a supplement? The answer is absolutely yes. Use a supplement, particularly if you're not in the sun and you don't drink milk, or you don't have any sources of fortified vitamin D in your diet. Take a supplement. Keep in mind that nutrition has to be consistent for it to work, so you're going to have to have cues to remind yourself to take your vitamin D. Maybe leave it on your kitchen counter. Maybe put it by your toothbrush. I've actually had patients who have taken their vitamin D bottle and taped it to the deodorant. Since you're not going to leave the house without using deodorant, this might be a way to remember. You have to do it on a regular basis for it to work.

Thank you very much, and go out and prevent cancer.

Nutrition and Digestive Health
Lecture 25

About 60–70 million people are affected by digestive diseases per year.

L et's look at the normal digestion process while considering the most common disorders. I had a patient who was lethargic. Despite eating large amounts of animal protein, he had iron deficiency anemia. It turned out this was due to high levels of pain medication, which altered his digestive tract. Nutrition is a key player when it comes to digestive health.

The upper digestive tract includes the mouth, esophagus, and stomach. Let's start with oral diseases. Saliva is required for digestion and for moisture. In conditions such as radiation for head and neck cancer, saliva can be compromised; that moisture must be replaced with moist foods. Dysphagia is a chronic disruption of the normal swallowing mechanism. To prevent aspiration of liquid foods, we can add thickeners to prevent them from leaving the mouth quickly.

Nutrition is a key player when it comes to digestive health.

Gastroesophageal reflux disease (GERD) is a condition where the acidified stomach contents reflux into the esophagus. Many causes of GERD include changes in the pressure of the lower esophageal sphincter. Managing GERD means reducing acid production and preventing reflux by consuming a low-fat diet and avoiding certain foods. Other lifestyle strategies include losing weight, getting regular physical activity, avoiding known gastric irritants, eating small meals, eating slowly, sleeping with the head of the bed elevated, and controlling your intake of aspirin or nonsteroidal anti-inflammatory drugs.

Antacids and medications designed to reduce acid production are popular, but any medication you take chronically may have a nutritional complication.

Now we get to the stomach, and to ulcer diseases. Ulcer symptoms include burning stomach pain, black tarry stools, nausea, vomiting, indigestion, heartburn, and weight loss. Ulcers can occur both in the stomach and in the small intestine. The dietary and nutritional management for both are similar. *H. pylori* is a bacterium that can cause ulcers. Sometimes ulcers can be secondary to other diseases. Diets can be supportive and aid in the healing process.

There are many diseases and conditions that affect the small and large intestine. Let's examine irritable bowel syndrome. Symptoms include abdominal pain, chronic diarrhea, and chronic constipation. The syndrome is caused by visceral hypersensitivity; another contributor is stress or chronic anxiety. Treatments include a lower- or higher-fiber diet, depending on symptoms; eliminating foods to which the patient is sensitive; and consuming probiotics.

Lactose intolerance is one of the most common digestive conditions and can affect people of all age groups. Symptoms include discomfort after consuming milk products, usually within a couple of hours. The intolerance is due to an insufficiency of lactase; it can also be caused by an infection or inflammation of the intestinal tract. Being somewhat deficient in lactase is normal; however, most people can tolerate up to 12 g (grams) of lactose per day.

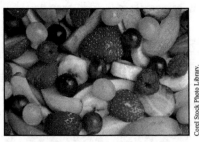

Celiac disease involves a sensitivity to gluten, which is a protein in grains such as wheat, barley, and rye. It is thought to be an autoimmune disorder. Symptoms may occur in the digestive tract or in other

You can increase your fiber intake by adding fruits, vegetables, nuts, and whole grains to your diet.

areas of the body. Some people are genetically predisposed to celiac disease. When individuals with celiac disease eat gluten, their immune systems attack, damage, and destroy the villi in the small intestine that help their body absorb nutrients. The treatment for celiac disease is to eat a gluten-free diet.

Diverticular disease is an inflammation of the diverticula in the intestinal tract. Symptoms include abdominal pain, particularly tenderness in the lower left side. To avoid this disease, eat whole grains and a lot of fruits and vegetables to avoid constipation. Antibiotics are one of the mainstay treatments for diverticulitis, to reduce the inflammation. Recovery would generally involve a low-residue diet as well.

Let's review some frequently asked questions. How do I increase the fiber in my diet gradually? Start with fruits, vegetables, nuts, whole grains, and high-fiber breakfast cereals.

What about fiber supplements? Be careful. Fiber can alter your body's ability to absorb many minerals. If you have constipation, make sure you are not dehydrated. ■

Suggested Reading

Duyff, *American Dietetic Association Complete Food and Nutrition Guide*, chap. 22.

Mahan and Stump, *Krause's Food, Nutrition, and Diet Therapy*, chaps. 30–31.

Questions to Consider

1. What digestive disorders have you experienced in your life? How have you dealt with them?

2. How has the study of various digestive disorders shown how disease often has a domino effect on our bodies?

Nutrition and Digestive Health
Lecture 25—Transcript

Greetings, and welcome back. I had a football player I was working with, and he was tired and lethargic, out of energy. I took his diet and he was a traditional American football player. He was a carnivore. As we explored some of his dietary habits and the medications he was taking, I looked at his blood work. He was profoundly anemic. He had iron deficiency anemia, despite eating large amounts of animal protein. Well, how did that happen? He had an alteration in his digestive tract because he was taking a lot of pain medication.

In this lecture, we're going to integrate the normal process of digestion, the way your body is supposed to behave, with the most common digestive disorders. Now, nutrition is a key player when it comes to discussing digestive health, and what we eat can make a difference. With many of the disorders we're going to look at, there may be no cure per se, but rather control through nutrition and dietary choices, lifestyle changes, and, again, possibly medication. I'm going to start out and orient you. We're going to divide the digestive tract into two sections, the upper GI and the lower GI. In the upper digestive tract, we're going to look at the mouth, the esophagus, and the stomach. So let's get started. Let's start taking a look at oral diseases.

Nutrition does begin in the mouth. We know that saliva is required for digestion and for moisture. In conditions such as radiation for head and neck cancer, saliva can be compromised. And the food must be moist because when you lose the natural ability of saliva to moisten food, you're going to have to replace that moisture with moist foods. This might include things like applesauce, soups, mashed potatoes with gravy, and yes, I did say "gravy," or margarine. What we're trying to do is integrate the disease with replacing some of those missed substances, like saliva, with moisture in the food.

What about dysphagia? Dysphagia occurs when there's a disruption of the normal swallowing mechanism. As food passes through the esophagus, there's a complex mechanism to make sure that the food is propelled into the esophagus, rather than into the trachea or the windpipe. Sometimes food accidentally makes its way to the trachea, probably due to an incomplete closure of the vocal chords. For most of us, this is occasional and it's uncomfortable, but it's the experience of choking on our food. When this becomes chronic, it's not the occasional episode, but when it becomes chronic, it is called "dsyphagia." It can occur when any step of the swallowing mechanism is disrupted. When the food ends up in the trachea, you're breathing in your food and aspiration pneumonia can occur, and it can be life-threatening.

Some of the most common causes would include stroke, head injury, and Parkinson's disease. Well, how does nutrition help here? Think about this. Liquid foods leave your mouth quickly. If the nervous system is disrupted, like in stroke, liquids are going to be the most commonly aspirated food. So what can we do to prevent that? Well, there are special thickeners that exist to thicken commonly enjoyed liquids, such as coffee, milk, and juice, without ruining the taste. Again, in health care, we always have partners, and in dysphagia, a speech therapist and a speech pathologist can assist in the swallowing mechanism and actually can help patients to develop positional changes, a change in the way their head is when they swallow, which can aid in the swallowing response.

After food reaches the stomach, it is acidified, and this is so key. We've covered this in the lecture on digestion. If the acidified stomach contents reflux or backwash into the esophagus, we have what is known as "gastroesophageal reflux disease," and you see this advertized in magazines and on television as "GERD." Now, your stomach is protected against acid, but the soft tissue of the esophagus has no such defense. You can experience a burning sensation in your chest that we call "heartburn." Actually, what it is is the acid that is backwashing into that soft tissue and causing pain and irritation. Many causes of GERD include changes in the pressure of the lower esophageal sphincter, known as "LES." Our bodies are designed with a series of one-way valves to help food go south, and the LES is one of the first valves that we encounter.

So an example here might be a hiatal hernia, where there are changes in that esophageal sphincter pressure. Normally, your stomach is below your diaphragm, but when it protrudes into the thoracic cavity, GERD can occur. There's less of the ability to keep that LES closed, and so there can be a leakage of stomach acid on a continual basis. This is because of the protrusion of a portion of the stomach into the thoracic cavity after passing through an opening in the diaphragm.

Sometimes an un-thought of consequence, or a cause of GERD, is obesity, particularly central obesity. Remember, that central obesity is the fat that accumulates in our abdomen. Another common cause, but uncommonly thought about, is your clothing. If you wear tight clothing around your midsection, or if you pull your belt tightly, you can put undue pressure on that LES and cause reflux. Smoking can alter LES pressure and also contribute to GERD, so again, we're talking about some environmental or lifestyle changes that you might want to have.

Managing GERD centers around reducing acid production and preventing reflux. It is usually recommended that individuals with GERD consume a low-fat meal, as it is thought that fat helps to delay gastric emptying time. If the food hangs around too long, you are more likely to have reflux. Although food affects each one of us differently, if you suffer from GERD, you may want to consider avoiding some of the following foods. Many of these recommended food omissions are due to either their effect on gastric secretions and/or LES. Common offenders include chocolate, onions, juice and carbonated beverages, peppers, mustard, tea, and real peppermint or spearmint. Think about this. Many people take peppermint candies in order to minimize GERD, and actually, if it's real peppermint, it may actually make it worse.

Coffee may or may not be a culprit. Although research has not shown that coffee is a risk factor for GERD, sufferers are often advised to avoid coffee consumption, primarily due to the amount of caffeine in coffee. Eating high-fiber bread rather than low-fiber white bread can significantly reduce the risk of reflux. Why is that? It's promoting that food leaving the stomach a little faster. Alcohol shows no real significant difference in GERD symptoms. However, many individuals will find if they have alcoholic beverages, they have enhanced symptoms, and the bottom line is if it bothers you, don't eat it or drink it.

Other lifestyle strategies to try for GERD include losing weight, regular physical activity, avoid the known gastric irritants, as well as those that bother you, eat small meals to reduce pressure on LES, eat slowly enough to allow adequate transit time for the food, sleep with the head of your bed elevated to keep the stomach contents where they belong in the stomach, particularly if you have hiatal hernia. And control your intake of aspirin or non-steroidal anti-inflammatory drugs. Well, what about medications? Are there medications that you can use? Certainly, antacids and medications designed to reduce acid production are popular, but I want you to think about this. Any medication you take chronically may have a nutritional complication.

In the case of antacids, buffering the stomach can reduce the acidification that actually does improve the bioavailability of thiamin and iron. Thiamin and iron must be acidified to be absorbed. Bacteria, also, that we all eat in our food are more likely to grow and survive in this more neutral or buffered pH. Some of the medications that are used actually have the potential to reduce the release of intrinsic factor, which is needed to unlock vitamin B_{12} from food. So again, any medication that you take chronically may have a nutritional complication.

We get to the stomach, and to ulcer diseases. Symptoms include burning stomach pain, black tarry stools, nausea, vomiting, indigestion, heartburn, and weight loss. Now, ulcers can occur both in the stomach and in the small intestine. However, the dietary and nutritional management for both are similar. So what causes ulcer disease? Well, *H. pylori* is a bacterium, and early in my clinical practice, ulcers were thought to be solely caused by stress or poor diet. As such, the thought was, we'll coat the stomach and protect it from acid. This diet was called the "sippy diet." It consisted of cream and milk, and as the science evolved, bacteria emerged as the major cause of ulcer disease, and it causes 90% of this disease.

Sometimes ulcers can be secondary to other diseases. For example, if a person needs to take non-steroidal anti-inflammatory drugs, say, for example, for significant arthritis, so arthritis may be the disease that now contributes to ulcers because of the role of these medications on stomach lining. Actually, what will happen is the lining of the stomach fails or weakens and allows the acid in the stomach to erode the lining, and that's actually what happened with my football player.

Treatment when it's *H. pylori* must include antibiotics and again, avoidance of medications that might contribute to the erosion of stomach lining. Now, certainly, diet can be supportive and aid in the healing process. Each patient has a very individual diet, but some nutritional choices that might improve this condition include avoid consuming large meals to reduce acid production. Consume soluble fiber that helps to normalize gastric emptying time. Soluble fiber also stimulates what is known as the production of short-chain fatty acids, which are associated with actually the regeneration of that damaged mucosa. Consuming omega-3 fatty acids and omega-6 fatty acids may also help to regenerate mucosal cells. Keep in mind that omega-3 fatty acids are most commonly associated with coldwater fish. Now, there may be some things to avoid. Peppers have been shown to increase acid secretions. Coffee and caffeine may also do that as well, but the bottom line is if it causes you individual distress, avoid it.

As we move on down the GI tract, we actually come to the lower GI system. There are many diseases and conditions that affect the small and large intestine. In this section, we're going to cover the following disorders, as they are often the most common, and they include irritable bowel syndrome, lactose intolerance, celiac disease, which sometimes is referred to as "gluten-induced enteropathy," and diverticular disease.

So let's examine irritable bowel. Some of the symptoms are abdominal pain, chronic diarrhea, or chronic constipation, and sometimes these are alternating, so you actually get a combination of both of them. Well, what causes it? If you're looking in the medical literature, the word that you're going to see is "visceral hypersensitivity," but sometimes I just refer to this as "fussy gut." You feel more discomfort with the presence of gas in your GI tract than normal. You feel more sensation associated with the presence of food in your intestine, so again, you actually have a hypersensitivity to food as it transverses through the intestinal tract. Certainly, individuals with irritable bowel can have altered intestinal motility. Sometimes it's faster, sometimes it's slower. They can also have the abnormal transit time of gas and stools. Sometimes it's fast, sometimes it's slow.

Another contributor to irritable bowel is stress or chronic anxiety, and so I would think in most of our lifestyles, we do have some degree of stress and anxiety. The problem is, as with many GI disorders, irritable bowel can oftentimes be confused with dietary or lactose intolerance. Celiac disease, again, intolerance to gluten in foods, may be confused with irritable bowel, or may be the actual cause of irritable bowel.

So what kinds of treatments exist for irritable bowel? Well, sometimes you can consume a lower fiber diet if diarrhea is the presenting symptom, and a higher fiber diet during periods of constipation. You eliminate the foods to which the patient is sensitive, and this comes up over and over again. If you think, well, every time I eat, fill in the blank, I end up having problems with my gut, then you might be sensitive to that food, just because you're you. And a way to manage this is you might want to think about keeping a food diary to track foods, along with symptoms, to see if you can figure out what's unique about you.

Certainly, things like probiotics, such as yogurt, might be helpful, and we cover that topic in another lecture. These are foods with healthy bacteria that can help to balance gut function and normalize bowel motility. In my practice, I find that a really very viable solution for many is to try probiotics. Certainly, since stress may be a cause, lifestyle changes might be recommended to lessen the stress. I have a lot of patients with irritable bowel who, for example, participate in yoga. Again, as with most chronic GI disorders, medications may be prescribed. I want you to think if a medication is prescribed, ask the question of your pharmacist, is there a nutritional consequence of this that I should be aware of?

What about lactose intolerance? This is one of the most common conditions and it can affect people of all age groups, but it is more common in African Americans. Now, what are the symptoms? Discomfort after consuming milk products, and it's usually within a couple of hours of consuming milk products, nausea, cramps, bloating, gas, and diarrhea. So physiologically, what causes this? Why do you have lactose intolerance? It is an insufficiency of lactase, and you remember from the lecture on carbohydrates, lactase in digestion is the enzyme that helps you to digest lactose. It can also be caused by an infection or an inflammation of the intestinal tract, or it can be secondary to another disease, including anything that's going to damage the villi in the small intestine, such as occurs in celiac or Crohn's disease. Remember that lactase enzymes are going to sit on the tip of the villi, the absorptive part of your small intestine, and if you have any damage to your small intestine, the lactase enzyme can temporarily go away.

What's the treatment? Being somewhat deficient in lactase is normal for most people. However, most of us can tolerate, even with mild lactose intolerance, up to a cup of milk or 12 grams of lactose per day. Research shows that avoiding milk will probably make individuals less tolerant to consuming milk products because the bacteria in the colon never learned to adapt to it efficiently. And again, when you demand that your body make lactase, your body's going to respond up to its biological capabilities.

There are some keys points here. You can buy reduced lactose products in the dairy section, or you can take over-the-counter lactase pills. They can be placed in the liquids to counteract the lactose before the consumption, so most symptoms are not felt, but timing is everything here. If you decide to take the lactase pill 20 minutes after you had milk, you've waited too long and that's actually too late. Those individuals avoiding milk may actually need to take a calcium supplement because remember, you've created a nutrient hole because you've eliminated a food group. Note that fermented products, such as yogurt, are better tolerated because they have the enzyme lactase in the food, and that's actually produced by wonderful probiotic bacteria.

What about celiac disease? Celiac disease patients are sensitive to gluten, which is a protein in grains such as wheat, barley, and rye. It is thought to be one of the autoimmune disorders. In fact, those with type 1 diabetes, another autoimmune disorder, are more likely to develop or have celiac disease. Some estimates indicate that celiac disease is under-diagnosed and the actual prevalence may be as high as 1 in 133 people. So this is one that if you have one of those things that we call "fussy gut," you may actually have undiagnosed celiac disease. Symptoms may occur in the digestive tract, or in other areas of the body. Infants and young children are more susceptible to the digestive symptoms. Adults may experience iron deficiency anemia, osteoporosis, and an actual skin condition called "dermatitis herpetiformis."

What causes it? Well, certainly we know that with celiac disease, there is a genetic predisposition. Prevalence is higher in relatives of persons with celiac disease, so if someone in your family has it, you have an increased likelihood because of the genetic predisposition. Consumption of foods containing wheat, barley, and rye causes irritation and discomfort. Actually, what the gluten does is it damages the villi in the small intestine. Now, studies show that oat consumption is a little bit more controversial. Some studies are going to suggest that, yes, if you consume oats, you may have some exacerbation of your gluten intolerance, and other studies say no. When individuals with celiac disease eat gluten, their immune systems attack, and damage, and destroy the villi in the small intestine that help their body to absorb nutrients. So again, remember, this is an autoimmune disorder.

For a true diagnosis, you have to have a biopsy of the small intestine to test for the presence of certain antibodies. But 50% of celiac patients, however, have few or no obvious symptoms. What's our recommended treatment here of celiac disease? It's 100% gluten-free diet adherence, and again, manufacturers have made this so much easier in the last few years. They've labeled products "gluten free," not just wheat free, but gluten free. If you're on this gluten-free diet, most major symptoms are going to disappear within two to eight weeks. What's happening is the villi in your small intestine are actually regenerating. Read labels to avoid things like wheat, rye, or barley. Check labels on seasoning and, oftentimes, you're going to have to actually call the food company for a clarification. Again, please remember, "wheat free" does not mean "gluten free."

Damage to the villi in the small intestine. This diet may make you deficient in other nutrients. So again, think about it this way. If I'm eliminating grains, I may be eliminating, for example, magnesium, and other minerals as well. So here are some strategies. Have adequate calcium and vitamin D in your diet to prevent osteoporosis and osteomalacia, which is also known as "adult rickets." You may need to increase the amount of iron in your diet to account for the exclusion of iron-fortified foods maybe with wheat, rye, or barley. Include folate-rich foods, such as fortified breakfast cereals. But again, remember, you want to stay away from those that are going to be made from suspect grains. So maybe you want to have a fortified rice breakfast cereal. And again, you could also go to green leafy vegetables as a source of folate-rich foods.

Because fatty acid malabsorption can cause a decrease in the absorption of fat-soluble vitamins, focus on foods rich in these nutrients, to include cantaloupe, carrots, nuts, and seeds, as tolerated. Some patients may find that a low-lactose diet might be useful in controlling symptoms at first. Keep in mind, once the GI tract returns to normal, though, you should always try and add back a little bit of lactose. So again, celiac is an example of a disease where, due to damage to your small intestine, you can develop temporary or secondary lactose intolerance.

What about diverticular disease? Diverticular disease, and diverticulitis, is actually an inflammation of the diverticulum, so we're going to explore that in a little bit more detail. Some symptoms are abdominal pain, particularly tenderness in the lower left side. What causes it? It's caused by the infection of the diverticula. What are diverticula? They're little outpoochings in the intestinal tract. So the lining of your intestinal tract is supposed to be smooth. When you have diverticular disease, you get a little bit of outpooching in the wall of that intestinal tract. As it outpooches, food can get trapped. It's often thought to be associated with constipation. So if you are constipated and you bear down or strain to have a bowel movement, the increased pressure in that intestinal wall can cause an outpooching in the intestinal wall.

This is oftentimes associated with our traditional American diet of highly processed foods. If you think, I really would like to prevent this disease, this is where eating whole grains and a lot of fruits and vegetables and the avoidance of constipation is really pretty key. Keep in mind we've talked about constipation in another lecture, but I'm going to remind you that constipation can be caused by inadequate fiber, inadequate hydration, and poor exercise habits. This diverticula then can oftentimes be obstructed by fecal matter, causing inflammation and pain. If it ruptures, it can actually spread bacteria into the peritoneal cavity, and cause a true bacterial infection.

What are the treatments? In the acute phase, the phase with significant amounts of pain, antibiotics are going to be one of the mainstay treatments for diverticulitis to reduce the inflammation. Oftentimes, as part of that recovery, you might want to begin with a low-residue diet, and keep in mind that residue means anything that is not completely digested. Certainly, fiber would contribute to residue, but other foods, such as milk, that are not completely digested may also contribute to residue and would be avoided on a low-residue diet. You may start out there, but then you're gradually going to return to a higher fiber diet to, again, prevent constipation.

This high-fiber diet may promote soft, bulky stools that require less straining. With less straining, there's lower intracolonic pressures, and for patients who didn't have a high-fiber diet before, please always know that you have to gradually increase the fiber in your diet. This is an example where you can't go from low fiber to high fiber because you can have significant GI upset. Certainly, ensure that there's an adequate amount of exercise and get adequate amounts of fluid to avoid that constipation. If you are sensitive or you experience pain with nuts and seeds, keep in mind they can get trapped in that diverticulum and cause inflammation or irritation. Avoid them if you are sensitive.

Now certainly, there are other GI disorders and so another frequently asked question, one that I hear quite often is, My daughter has been recently diagnosed with Crohn's disease. What is it, and where can I find out more about it? Keep in mind when you search the internet that there can be unbelievably reliable sources, and some, not so much. What is Crohn's disease? Crohn's disease is an inflammatory bowel disease. In Crohn's disease, all of the multiple layers of the intestinal tract become inflamed. As such, the intestinal wall becomes damaged, and also causes the malabsorption of vital nutrients, along with significant diarrhea. Here's an example where diet is supportive, but it's not curative. Many people who have Crohn's disease believe that if they follow a prescribed diet that that's going to cure Crohn's, but unfortunately I think that we are years away from a cure. To find out details about Crohn's and other digestive related diseases, among your best sources on the web is the National Institute of Diabetes and Digestive and Kidney Diseases. It's going to give you details about the disease, including symptoms, how it's treated, and other useful information. Another concern about Crohn's disease is as the intestinal wall becomes damaged, and becomes inflamed, oftentimes there is a narrowing of that intestinal lumen, or tube, and oftentimes individuals will have to have bowel resections, or they may not be able to tolerate high fiber foods. This is a great example where you must partner with your physician. And again with Crohn's as well as with other kinds of GI disorders, oftentimes medications are going to be part of the mainstay of treatment.

Another frequently asked question is, I've always heard that I need to increase the fiber in my diet, and to do so gradually, but how do I do this? Well, certainly, fruits and vegetables are an easy fix, and here's an example. If you normally have orange juice in the morning, maybe what you want to do is have a sliced whole orange. If you're hard-pressed to give up that orange juice in the morning, maybe purchase one with higher pulp content. Fruits and vegetables are going to be an easy way to add more fiber to your diet. Another thing that you can do is choose high-fiber breakfast cereals. But again, because they have so much fiber per serving, here's a tip for you. Take your regular breakfast cereal, the one that you've grown up with and love, and you add a couple of tablespoons of the high-fiber breakfast cereal. You're enriching it with fiber, but you're not going from 0 to 60 in your fiber intake. As your body becomes accustomed to it, every few days, add just a few more tablespoons. Maybe you get to a point where you're looking at half of your regular cereal and half of your high fiber one.

Keep in mind that nuts are also going to be a great source of fiber. Whole grains are a great source of fiber. But bodies need time to adapt, so one of the biggest barriers I see in clinical practice is individuals who go too quickly. They switch from their regular morning breakfast cereal to a high-fiber version. They're on it for a day or two. They have significant GI upset and they think, my gut can't tolerate this. My response is, yes, it can, but you gave it too much too quickly. Again, remember your digestive tract is this wonderful, complex machinery, but it needs time to adapt to something new.

A companion question to that is, what about fiber supplements? Aren't fiber supplements beneficial? Can't I just go to a pill? I always say, be careful with the fiber supplements. Keep in mind, a lot of fiber at a particular meal, and particularly in a supplement form, can alter your body's ability to absorb many minerals, so that would be the first concern that I would have. If you're using a fiber supplement for constipation, have you explored the other causes of constipation? Are you dehydrated? What is the color of your urine? Remember, if your urine looks like pale lemonade, you're probably hydrated. If it looks like apple juice, you're not. The real tragedy that I see is individuals can take a fiber supplement without adequate amounts of fluid, and actually make their constipation worse.

Also, you want to think about the type of fiber supplement. If you're really trying to treat constipation, bran is going to be better than a commercially available supplement that has psyllium in it. Keep in mind bran is going to be great. You can go to your health food store and buy bran very inexpensively, and you could add bran to applesauce. You can even add bran to mashed potatoes. But remember, go slowly for the best GI outcome.

Thank you very much.

Prebiotics and Probiotics in Your Diet
Lecture 26

Probiotics are the healthy bacteria found in foods and, now, as food additives or in functional foods. Prebiotics are the fuel that feeds probiotics.

Let's explore the exciting new arena of pre- and probiotics. Almost 30 years ago in my clinical practice, we had a significant number of tube-fed patients developing diarrhea. We added yogurt to their diet to blunt the diarrhea, though at the time we did not know why it worked. This lecture is going to explore the science of prebiotics and probiotics, as well as supplements that can help maintain good intestinal health.

Probiotics are healthy bacteria. They are found in foods and, now, as food additives or in functional foods. Examples include fermented foods like yogurt and soy products, some juices, and pickles and sauerkraut. Élie Metchnikoff first observed, in the early 1900s, that Bulgarian peasants who consumed fermented food and milk products lived longer and healthier lives. Probiotics are defined by the World Health Organization and the Food and Agriculture Organization as live microorganisms that, in adequate amounts, confer a health benefit. There is no true requirement for the amount of probiotic needed, because it can autopopulate in your gut.

Prebiotics feed the probiotics. Fiber compounds are the most significant prebiotics—specifically, inulin and its by-products, fructo-oligosaccharides and galacto-oligosaccharides. Major food sources of fructo-oligosaccharides include chicory root, Jerusalem artichoke, leeks, and onions. High-fiber breakfast cereals and bars use chicory root as a fiber source. Fructo-oligosaccharides are also being added to liquid nutritional meal replacements. Doses of above 15 g of prebiotics can cause gastric upset.

Let's take a look at the gut environment. At birth, your gut is sterile. It is colonized by bacteria, depending on the mode of feeding. The oligosaccharides from breast milk function as a prebiotic. The breast milk itself contains probiotic bacteria that support immune function. The intestinal tract is also involved in the immune response through gut-associated lymphoid tissue.

Health claims are being made for prebiotics. Some studies suggest an improvement in blood sugar and blood cholesterol, but results are not consistent. Other claims include improved magnesium absorption and a slight increase in copper absorption. Prebiotics may also reduce atopic dermatitis, as well as infections in the first 2 years of life.

In general, probiotics can assist in optimizing health.

In general, probiotics can assist in optimizing health. *Lactobacillus acidophilus*–cultured dairy products can reduce vaginal yeast infections. Probiotics may prevent sexually transmitted diseases via changes in vaginal pH. *Lactobacillus* may also aid in the reduction of cholesterol.

Probiotics have recently been associated with a reduction of obesity in pregnant mothers. In those with lactose intolerance, *Lactobacillus* helps to provide an easily digested, high-calcium dairy product. *Lactobacillus acidophilus* and other probiotics have been shown to reduce diarrhea and other digestive diseases.

Supplements can create challenges. Concerns include whether they can be contaminated, the amount of probiotic needed, issues of probiotic viability, whether these products survive in stomach acid, and avoiding competing pathogenics. Although not all probiotics can withstand the very low pH in stomach acid, some produce significant amounts of lactic acid, which may inhibit the growth of unfriendly bacteria.

Are probiotics always safe? They are generally regarded as safe; however, those with altered immune systems should be cautious of products containing probiotics.

If you get enough fiber in your diet, then you are getting enough prebiotics. As for probiotics, consider adding some fermented foods to your diet.

Let's review some frequently asked questions. What happens if we do not consume probiotics or prebiotics? Our guts will be more nutritionally challenged.

Exposure to moisture may reduce the effectiveness of probiotics, but isn't our digestive tract full of moisture? Yes, but what you want to avoid is chronic exposure of the supplements to moisture, as in your bathroom or car.

Are there certain times in the life cycle that pre- and probiotics are important? Once antibiotics are used, pre- and probiotics are needed to repopulate the gut.

Should I add probiotic and prebiotic supplements to my children's or parents' diet? Unless they have an unusual gut disease, these are safe.

If I do not like yogurt or fiber, can I just take a pill? That is an option, but it is always best to eat whole foods. ∎

Suggested Reading

Huffnagle and Wernick, *The Probiotics Revolution*.

Questions to Consider

1. What examples of probiotics and prebiotics do you already incorporate in your diet?

2. How do cultural differences affect our food choices?

Prebiotics and Probiotics in Your Diet
Lecture 26—Transcript

Hello, and welcome. My clinical practice dates back almost 30 years. In the beginning of my clinical practice, I worked at Tulane University Medical Center in New Orleans, and we had a significant number of tube-fed patients, patients who couldn't eat voluntarily on their own. And what we noticed is that the longer they were tube-fed, the more likely they were to develop diarrhea. One of the strategies that we implemented was adding yogurt to this tube feeding to blunt the diarrhea. We didn't really know why it worked, but it worked. And so now, as we fast-forward, we have this whole new exciting arena of pre- and probiotics that we're going to explore.

It has been said that our body is formed around our gut. As such, think about your intestinal tract as the body's gatekeeper. This intricate balance of good and bad bacteria, healthy intestinal tissue, and optimal diet can keep the gut function normal, as well as confer some additional health benefits. Well, this lecture is going to explore the science of prebiotics and probiotics, as well as supplements that can help maintain good intestinal health. Let's start with some definitions.

What is a probiotic? Simply stated, a probiotic is healthy bacteria. It is found in foods and, now, as food additives or in functional foods. Examples of food sources containing probiotics are fermented foods, such as yogurt, yogurt products like kefir. However, watch out, chocolate lovers. Some chocolate yogurts are pasteurized. That pasteurization process is high heat, and it kills the probiotics. These are live cultures and are killed with heat. Other fermented products include soy products like tempeh and miso, and some soy beverages. Some juices, pickles, and sauerkraut are also fermented products, and therefore would contain some probiotics.

In probiotic foods and supplements, the bacteria might have been originally present, or they may have been added during the preparation and production. Another way of looking at probiotic is that it means prolife. The necessity of these compounds was first identified by Dr Élie Metchnikoff, a Nobel Prize-winning scientist in the early 1900s. Dr Metchnikoff observed that Bulgarian peasants who consumed fermented food and milk products lived longer and healthier lives. Probiotics, as a definition, are defined by the World Health Organization and the Food and Agriculture Organization as live microorganisms. That's a key point. Live microorganisms, which, when administered in adequate amounts, confer a health benefit on the host. Although an accepted definition exists, there are no national standards for identifying the level of active probiotic in foods or supplements.

Also, there is no true requirement for the amount of probiotic needed when this compound is found in food. Little concern exists regarding the amounts needed because, remember, these are live organisms and once they are in your gut, can autopopulate and live there very happily on their own. Is this just a passing fad, or is this the fountain of digestive health and wellness? Well, let's take a look at the types of probiotics. In general, they are bacteria and yeast. Two major bacteria types include *lactobacillus*, and keep in mind, *lactobacillus* is the name of the central organism, but there are multiple species, and you might be familiar with *acidophilus* as a *lactobacillus* culture. *Bifidobacterium* is the general name, with *bifidus* being the particular strain that we're looking at.

The type of bacteria confers the function and benefit, so not all bacteria is going to have the identical function. Some bacterial strains may confer immune protection. Others may promote optimal gut function or regularity. Another probiotic type is yeast, with a major type being *saccharomyces boulardii*, and again, this is a probiotic yeast. Sometimes you hear it referred to as "nutritional yeast." But because these organisms are live, we have to feed these bacteria, and probiotics rely on the fuel provided in the diet. Now, I want you to think about this for a second. We can either have a really healthy diet, with adequate amounts of great food for the bacteria, or we can have a highly processed diet, and again, not going to provide adequate amounts of food for the bacteria.

The fuel that feeds the probiotics is called "prebiotics," and as a definition, it is non-digestible food components that support the growth or activity of probiotics. Simply put, prebiotics are the food for friendly bacteria. Fiber compounds are the most significant prebiotics. Specifically, inulin—and don't confuse that with insulin, which is a hormone—is a type of fiber and its byproduct, fructo-oligosaccharides, FOS, and galacto-oligosaccharides, GOS.

Now, let's pause for a second and define these terms. In the carbohydrate lecture, we talked about mono- and disaccharides, one or two glucose units, and then we jumped to polysaccharides, 20 or more glucose units. Well, there's an intermediate called "oligosaccharides," and these are 8 to 10 carbohydrate units. So fructo-oligosaccharide would be a compound, predominantly made of fructose, with 8 to 10 carbohydrate units in that chain.

The major food sources of inulin and its metabolite, fructo-oligosaccharides, in the American diet include foods maybe that you don't normally consume, things like chicory root, Jerusalem artichoke, leeks, and onions. The amount of inulin and fructo-oligosaccharide in chicory root, for example, is there's 24 grams of inulin and 43 grams of fructo-oligosaccharides in a 3 ounce serving. Well, here's the key point. If you look now at a lot of high-fiber breakfast cereals and bars, they are using chicory root as the fiber source. So when they use chicory root, they are adding essentially inulin and fructo-oligosaccharides to that food, without naming them. They're just talking about the chicory root, and you'll see this popping up in grocery stores.

Fructo-oligosaccharides are also being added to liquid nutritional meal replacements, such as Ensure. So if you remember back to my example about my tube-fed patient, one of the challenges was, in the early days of tube-feeding, we didn't know anything about fructo-oligosaccharides. We had no clue. Now, when fructo-oligosaccharides are added to these liquid nutritional meal replacements, some of which you drink orally, some of which are in tube-feeding, you can now blunt or reduce the incident of diarrhea by consuming these products that have FOS added to them.

As with almost everything in clinical nutrition, more is not better. Doses of above 15 grams of these prebiotics can cause gastric upset, which should make sense because these are basically fiber-containing foods. So together, this marriage of pre- and probiotics work to fuel this wonderful complex called a "symbiotic." They work synergistically together to optimize gut function. So now let's take a look at the gut environment.

At birth, your gut is sterile. There is no bacteria in your gut. It is colonized by bacteria, depending on the mode of feeding. Well, breast milk contains oligosaccharides, so once again, Mother Nature steps in and provides us with the nutrition that we need. The oligosaccharides from breast milk function as a prebiotic. The breast milk itself contains probiotic bacteria that can help to confer some of the benefits that we associate with breast feeding. These bacteria support the immune function through a unique and wonderful physiological response.

The intestinal tract is also involved in the immune response, through gut associated lymphoid tissue, which is also known as "GALT." Large areas of lymphoid tissues are found in the gut in the Peyer's patches, and we learned a little bit about these in the lecture on digestion. The intestinal tract represents a portion of the immune system, so how many of you have ever thought, I wonder where my immune system resides? Well, a good percentage of that is going to reside in your intestinal tract. Does that make sense? If our bodies are wrapped around our gut, we need to have an immune defense system in our intestinal tract to prevent bacterial invasion to our blood supply. Also, it aids in the prevention of food-borne illnesses.

In gut injury or infection, dangerous or unhealthy pathogenic bacteria can translocate. What does that mean? It means that these bacteria or their toxins can leave the small intestine and cross into the blood supply, causing blood-borne infections. Some studies suggest that even healthy bacteria may be able to translocate. So you better check with your health-care provider if you've had a significant bowel injury or surgery because any bacterial translocation, good or bad, that's not supposed to end up in the blood supply, can make you ill. Bacterial translocation is considered to be a major cause of infection, particularly in an ill or hospitalized patient.

Now we've got health claims that are being made for prebiotics. Some studies suggest an improvement in blood sugar and blood cholesterol, but results are not consistent. Why might that be? Why aren't we always going to have consistent results when we start to talk about some of these research studies? Well, part of that is because we're all not identical twins, and we're all going to have unique physiological responses. The other reasons why we're not seeing consistent results are because the science of pre- and probiotics is relatively new. Improved magnesium absorption is also being claimed, along with a slight increase in copper absorption. However, improved mineral absorption really is not a valid reason for taking prebiotics. Again, I think what ends up happening is that as the science emerges, marketing jumps on the nutritional bandwagon and now we're going to have a lot of different products on the market, claiming pre- and probiotic benefits.

Prebiotics may also reduce atopic dermatitis, as well as infections in the first two years of life. Now, why would that make sense? A nice little study was done, taking a look at two groups of infants with a parental history of allergies, who were randomized to two groups. One group got prebiotics and the other did not. Those in the intervention group, those receiving the prebiotics, had significantly less dermatitis (skin irritation) and fewer infections. The benefits extended beyond the length of the intervention. Now, why might that be? Keep in mind these are live organisms, and the gut can colonize good bacteria, and that's the plausible explanation. The reason why the benefits continued beyond the study period was because the gut had colonized these good bacteria, set up shop, and they were growing in the small intestine.

What does the science say about probiotics? In general, probiotics can assist in optimizing health. *Lactobacillus acidophilus* is one of the *lactobacillus* strains that has beneficial effects. Some evidence suggests that *lactobacillus acidophilus* cultured dairy products, including sweet *acidophilus* milk and yogurt, can reduce vaginal yeast infections. Other studies suggest that probiotics may actually prevent sexually transmitted diseases via changes in the vaginal pH. Now, I probably would not suggest that that would be your only protection against sexually transmitted diseases. I don't think I'd hang my hat completely on pre- or probiotics.

Lactobacillus may also aid in the reduction of cholesterol. In a study done with one cup of yogurt with active cultures, or a placebo, individuals consuming probiotic-rich foods showed a 2.9% reduction in cholesterol. The mode of action here appears to be inhibition of the cholesterol-producing enzyme. Probiotics have recently been associated with a reduction of obesity in pregnant mothers after they receive probiotics during the first trimester of pregnancy. Approximately 25% of those receiving probiotics develop central obesity, compared to a higher percentage of those who received diet advice alone. This was presented at the European Society for Obesity, and this is the first study suggesting an association between probiotic use and body fat management. Now, again, this science is in its infancy, so we cannot make the quantum leap to say that if you're going to reduce body fat, everybody should be using probiotic-rich foods.

Major benefits of the *lactobacillus* organism for digestive health are relatively well known, and in those with lactose intolerance, the inability to digest lactose (milk sugar). Up to 50% of the lactose in fermented milk is actually digested by the lactase that is produced by the *lactobacillus* organism, providing an easily digested, high-calcium dairy product for those who struggle with lactose intolerance. One of the original review studies with *lactobacillus acidophilus* and other probiotics suggested that this family of probiotics has been shown to reduce diarrhea and other digestive diseases. The proposed mechanism is that these bacteria reduce the pH of the gut and crowd out pathogenic bacteria. So they prevent that translocation. They prevent some of the concerns that are associated with these pathogenic bacteria.

As such, some studies suggest, although not all, that probiotics may actually decrease the symptoms associated with traveler's diarrhea, irritable bowel, and even Crohn's disease. A recent meta-analysis indicated that probiotic therapy can significantly reduce the bloating associated with irritable bowel, and improve overall symptoms of inflammatory bowel disease. Here's a tip for you. For many of the women that I deal with that are struggling with IBS-like symptoms, the addition of a probiotic in my experience reduces that bloating by up to 40%, so it's really a great and very healthy strategy to take.

What about antibiotic-associated diarrhea? Think back to all my folks that were tube-fed at Tulane. One of the reasons why everybody developed diarrhea was because the products didn't have the wonderful prebiotics of fructo-oligosaccharides. The other reason was that everybody was on antibiotic therapy. So if you're taking antibiotics, keep in mind that antibiotics kill all bacteria, and if indeed you're given probiotics, it can reduce the severity and the intensity of the diarrhea. I'm going to say that again. Antibiotics kill all bacteria, and probiotics can repopulate the gut with healthy bacteria.

I'm going to caution you here. Think about taking your antibiotic and your probiotic at the same time. It's probably not how you want to time them, because if indeed I'm taking a medication that's going to kill bacteria, I don't want to take my probiotic, so spread those out. Well, you know how it goes. If we get a little bit of good press on these pre- and probiotics, now we enter into the supplement world, and supplements can create challenges. Keep in mind all of the studies that have been done have been done on whole foods. So when we talk about supplements, we have to remember purity and standardization remain issues, as they do for other supplements.

Currently, the issues associated with probiotic supplements include, could they be contaminated with other less desirable organisms? There's certainly disagreement on the amount of probiotic needed. Some authorities recommend at least 1 billion organisms a day, and I know that sounds huge, but we have trillions of bacteria in our digestive tract. A recent analysis showed that only 8 out of 13 products claiming to be probiotics listed probiotics on their label. Certainly, we have to be concerned about the issues of probiotic viability, and what does that mean? As opposed to other supplements, probiotics are live and are not going to survive harsh conditions. So one of the things that you can do is to refrigerate these products, and it may prolong the life. Again, we're trying to reduce their exposure to high temperatures. Exposure to moisture, like in your bathroom, may reduce the effectiveness of these products.

We also have to consider, will these products survive in stomach acid? The avoidance of competing pathogenics are key concerns in probiotic supplements. Although not all probiotics can withstand that very low pH in stomach acid, there may be still some benefit from them. Some of the bacteria species that do not survive stomach acid produce by themselves significant amounts of lactic acid, which may inhibit the growth of unfriendly bacteria, which is a really good thing. So again, it may not be the probiotic itself. It's the byproduct, in this case, lactic acid. We have to ask the question, are probiotics always safe? The key point here is gut integrity. Damage to the gut wall can allow any bacteria to translocate. However, I'm going to make my own comment here, the long positive history with probiotics in food have allowed them to be granted what is called "GRAS" status, meaning generally regarded as safe.

As we have seen, probiotics can assist in optimizing good health. However, some studies suggest that those with an altered immune system should be cautious of products containing probiotics. Clearly, more research needs to be conducted to find both additional benefits, and possible concerns with their use. Keep in mind our bodies like to go down the middle of the road, and probiotic foods are very beneficial. The question is, what about probiotic supplements? So where does this leave us regarding probiotics and prebiotics in the American diet?

First and foremost, if you get enough fiber in your diet, then you are getting enough prebiotics. Certainly, if you're eating fiber-enriched foods, foods with chicory, inulin, you're certainly getting adequate amounts of prebiotics. Keep in mind, though, vary your fiber sources and just don't label-read for chicory root. As for probiotics, consider adding some fermented foods to your diet. One of my favorite suggestions is to use Greek yogurt to replace sour cream in recipes, from dips to toppings, to baked goods, and even beef stroganoff. The key, however, is not to boil it. So if you're making a wonderful beef stroganoff, add the Greek yogurt at the end of the cooking period, not at the beginning of the cooking period.

Now we come to frequently asked questions. What happens if we don't consume probiotics or prebiotics? Is this detrimental to our health? Well, historically, people always had a source of this nutrient. Certainly, throughout time, when we ate more whole foods with fiber, and isn't that the key? It's the whole foods with fiber and some fermented products. We had exposure to a wide variety of pre- and probiotics. But have we moved away from this as an American culture? The answer is yes. The more highly processed the food becomes, the more hands that touch it along the way, that means we're actually removing some of the fiber, adding more sugars and fats, and reducing even the prebiotic content of our diet. Certainly, by making the switch in the American diet to more convenient and fast foods, we have now made our guts more nutritionally challenged.

Another question: You said that exposure to moisture may reduce the effectiveness of probiotics, but isn't our digestive tract full of moisture? Well, yes, that's absolutely true, but what we're looking at is chronic exposure of the supplements to moisture, like in your bathroom. If you're transporting probiotic supplements back and forth to work, the heat in your car, and the moisture in your car would also be very detrimental. Well, are there certain times in the life cycle that pre- and probiotics are important? What about illness, pregnancy, times of stress, times of unusually great physical activity? Well, the major reason why individuals get gut challenged is antibiotics, and the major reason why individuals end up with this imbalanced bacterial complement, again, is antibiotic therapy. It doesn't mean that you can eliminate antibiotics from your repertoire of treating disease, but you have to be conscious that once I introduce antibiotics, once antibiotics are part of my medical treatment, I'm going to have to make sure that I repopulate my gut with what it needs.

You could start off by just having additional yogurt when you're on antibiotics. You could have some additional fiber when your gut's a little bit resolved from that antibiotic therapy. Keep in mind, there's a famous way that we always treated antibiotic diarrhea, and it was called the "BRAT diet," and it was bananas, rice, applesauce, some people say tea, others say toast. I'm going to modify that for you and call it the "BRAY diet," and I'm going to say bananas, rice, applesauce, and add some yogurt. Now we've got again a little bit of fiber in the bananas and the applesauce. We've got some carbohydrate and lo and behold, we've now introduced a probiotic into the mix.

Should I add probiotic and prebiotic supplements to my children's diet? What about my aging parents? Unless there is an unusual gut disease, I would say probiotics are safe, and some cultures add yogurt to the diet of infants as one of the first foods given. Keep in mind breast milk has not only a prebiotic in the fructo-oligosaccharides, but it also has probiotics in it. So the first food that we're feeding babies, breast milk, is also going to be a great source of pre- and probiotics. As for aging parents, the same recommendation holds true. Fermented foods are always going to be a good idea, again, with some gentle sources of fiber.

Another question. I'll be traveling to some countries where I have to drink bottled water. Would eating the local yogurt help me to avoid traveler's diarrhea? Possibly, but I don't think I would risk a water-borne illness, such as a parasitic infection, and think that a probiotic will ride on its white horse to save you. You have to have common sense that prevails. But I would encourage you that if you're traveling, and you're in a foreign country, one of the key things that I would like you to think about is, can I try some of the local yogurts? That would be a great way of introducing some wonderful prebiotics and probiotics into your diet.

In many foreign countries, particularly when you travel to more remote regions, they're still eating a whole food diet, so I think the challenge is that when you eat a whole food diet, lots of fresh fruits and vegetables, adding in some fermented foods, is going to be your best defense against these chronic food-borne infections.

The other question that I get on a repeat basis is, well, I don't like yogurt and I don't really want to eat fiber, so what do I do? Can't I just take a pill? Certainly, throughout these series of lectures, we're making the case, we're laying the framework, for whole food is always going to prevail. Maybe you don't like yogurt, but could you eat a different fermented food? Could you have a soy drink that's fermented? Could you try miso or tempeh or some other fermented foods? Maybe if you're from the part of the country that I am, where sauerkraut is really very popular, maybe it's not yogurt, but put sauerkraut on your very lean or low-fat hot dog when you're grilling at home. There's lots of ways of introducing these.

I think the common sense is don't always think pill. We've got a lot of issues with dietary supplements in this country and again, with probiotics, just like every other supplement that's out there, we've got challenges that make that not the first choice. It is a choice, but not necessarily the best choice. Keep in mind common sense prevails. Mother Nature laid the framework by putting all these wonderful things in breast milk, and it's our job to make sure that we continue on this great path to optimal health.

Thank you very much.

Food Safety—It's in Your Hands
Lecture 27

Each year in the United States, food-borne illnesses affect 76 million people. These illnesses can be prevented to a certain extent by the consumer.

Foods become contaminated by 3 major methods: biological, chemical, or physical. Biological food contamination mainly occurs during the processing and preparation of foods. These problems may be traced to food preparers not washing their hands or not changing latex gloves when preparing different foods. Cutting boards can also be a source. More than 90% of all food-borne illnesses are caused by bacteria; of the bacteria we consume, only about 4% are pathogenic bacteria that can cause food-borne illnesses with gastrointestinal consequences. Common pathogenic bacteria include *Salmonella, Listeria, Shigella, E. coli, Campylobacter jejuni, Staph. aureus,* and *Clostridium botulinum.*

More than 90% of all food-borne illnesses are caused by bacteria.

Chemical food contamination can be a cause of illness. Chemical cross-contamination can be reduced by diligent washing. Skins of fruits and vegetables can become broken and contaminated with pesticides or other agricultural chemicals. Plant and animal toxins can also cause chemical contamination.

What about physical cross-contamination? This happens when foreign material, such as glass, bone, metal, or plastic, ends up in food. This is usually the result of an accident in a food production facility.

Certain populations experience more severe symptoms and are at higher risk for contracting a food-borne illness. These include infants and very young children, individuals greater than 65 years old, individuals with a compromised immune system or chronic illness, and pregnant women. The usual symptoms of food-borne illness are diarrhea, abdominal cramping, chills, fever, vomiting, and dehydration.

The United States has food safety regulating agencies at the federal, state, and local levels. Once an illness develops, a local health agency is usually the first to respond. If it looks like it is an epidemic, state and federal agencies become involved, if necessary. At the federal level, there are 3 agencies involved: the Centers for Disease Control and Prevention, the Food and Drug Administration, and the USDA Food Safety Inspection Service. There is also a federal system called Hazard Analysis Critical Control Point, designed to keep our food supply safe.

What about prevention methods? The agencies' roles include developing legislation to regulate the safety of food processing and handling. Consumer behaviors that influence food safety include hand washing, drying hands with a paper towel, keeping food temperature away from the danger zone, thawing food properly, cooking foods to the appropriate internal temperature, discarding any food that is questionable, and separating raw meat utensils from other foods and utensils. People do not realize the importance of food safety in power outages and flooding. The USDA has useful emergency preparedness fact sheets on its website.

Cook foods to their appropriate internal temperature. You can use a kitchen thermometer to determine the internal temperature.

- Ground meats (beef, hamburger): 160°F.

- Beefsteaks: at least 145°F.

- Pork: 160°F.

- Poultry: 180°F.

- Eggs (casseroles): 160°F.

Let's review some frequently asked questions. How do I know the difference between symptoms of a food-borne illness and stomach flu? It is hard to know, because the symptoms are similar. If you ate at a picnic or an unknown restaurant, it might be food borne.

Can you leave a frozen lunch on your desk for a couple of hours? Consider using a thermometer to check the internal temperature—or refrigerate it.

What can I do to keep school lunches safe? Freeze your juice boxes or water bottles and use them as cold packs.

How can I tell if a weather emergency shut off my freezer when I was away from home? Put an ice cube in a plastic container in the freezer. If it has melted and reformed, the freezer was off.

Is it bad to put hot food right into the refrigerator? No, most hot foods should go straight into the refrigerator.

What can I do if my child does not like to wash her hands in hot water? Use slightly cooler water and find other incentives, like singing songs or rewarding her with stickers. ■

Suggested Reading

Brown, A., *Understanding Food*, chaps. 3, 27.

Brown, J., *Nutrition Now*, unit 32.

Questions to Consider

1. What changes will you make in your food preparation habits to ensure safety?

2. Considering your geographic location, local climate, access to food and other supplies, and other circumstances, when might you experience situations that would require emergency preparedness?

Food Safety—It's in Your Hands
Lecture 27—Transcript

Welcome back. Well, we've all seen the headlines, tainted peanut butter, *E-coli* infected spinach or apple juice or hamburger, salmonella in peppers and tomatoes. What will happen next? Well, in this lecture on food safety, we're going to cover some very important key points on how we keep our food supply safe and what our role is as consumers.

Although the United States' food supply is regarding as one of the safest in the world, there are still concerns with food products becoming contaminated, as evidenced by the recent outbreaks. So what kind of protections do we have and what information do we know about food safety? Well, the Centers for Disease Control and Prevention, the CDC, estimates that each year in the United States, food-borne illnesses cause sickness in 76 million people. I want you to think about that for a second. We are always concerned about the new pandemic, whether it's avian flu or swine flu, but this is a real and tangible threat to the American health. There is sickness in 76 million people, and it results in approximately 325,000 hospitalizations, and over 5000 deaths. These food-borne illnesses can be caused by numerous factors, and can be prevented to a certain extent by the consumer. We all have a role in food safety.

We need to know not only about making good food choices, but also about preparing, handling, and storing food carefully. We all have our own family ways of managing food, whether it's preparing, handling, or storing food, and sometimes we might be the responsible culprit in the food poisoning incident. This lecture is going to help to keep you aware of the food that you are consuming by introducing you to food contamination methods. How do we get ill? What are the consequences, the signs, and the symptoms? Who regulates this for us? Who are our regulating agencies? Probably, most importantly, how do we prevent this? So let's explore how foods become contaminated.

We've got three major methods. It can be biological, chemical, and physical. Certainly, most of us think about the biological methods of food contamination as probably the most common. It mainly occurs during the processing and the preparation of foods onsite. These problems may be traced to food preparers not washing their hands, a very, very common cause of food poisoning, or not changing latex gloves when preparing different foods. So that means that someone may mix ground beef with latex gloves and really not think about the fact that now they're cutting tomatoes. So it can be not changing latex gloves in between different stops in the food supply chain.

Certainly, cutting boards can be a source as well, such as using a cutting board for meat or fish and then jumping to preparing raw or uncooked vegetables without washing the cutting board or using a different one. Certainly, you can get colored cutting boards and as a home strategy, you can use one just for meat, maybe red, and then the green for produce, and don't allow for that cross-contamination. Certainly, under biological methods, bacteria, moulds, viruses, and even parasites can exist in the food supply. Now, obviously, these are very small microorganisms that you may not be able to see.

Bacteria are the common cause of food-borne illness. It can enter the food supply during different stages of the processing, and most of it is killed or inactivated by adequate cooling or cooking procedures. So sometimes just being respectful of temperature guidelines can oftentimes minimize your risk of developing a food-borne illness. More than 90% of all food-borne illnesses are caused by bacteria, and of the bacteria that we consume, only about 4% are pathogenic. The remaining 96% are harmless. Keep in mind that this is oftentimes what we call the "probiotics." It can be used to produce items like cheese, yogurt, sour cream, fermented foods, such as pickles, sauerkraut, and some soy products. We've talked a little bit before about helpful bacteria, but now we need to look at the evil demons of pathogenic bacteria.

Pathogenic bacteria can cause food-borne illnesses with gastrointestinal consequences. Chances are if you're listening to this lecture, you've experienced food poisoning in the past, and so you have an up close and personal relationship with the gastrointestinal consequences. The infections of the majority of food-borne illnesses are ingesting harmful bacteria that grow in your intestine, replicate, and create the infection. So what are the common ones? *Salmonella* can contaminate food and water. Probably poultry products and eggs are where most people are going to think of with *salmonella*, but it's simple things like stuffing birds at Thanksgiving and not cooking to the proper internal temperature. Remember, oftentimes respecting those temperature gradients can be enough to prevent food-borne illnesses. So one tip that I'm going to give you is get a thermometer. You can't guess that internal temperature. You must measure internal temperature.

Certainly, when I was growing up, I had pet turtles and I remember my mother saying, "wash your hands, wash your hands." And yes, even pets can be a source of food-borne illnesses if you don't wash your hands.

Listeria is one of these bacteria that can survive a wide variety of pH. It also has the ability to grow in temperatures ranging from 39°F to 111°F, so what does that mean about the temperature gradient? It means the food has to be lower than 39°F, and if you're cooking it, it has to have a higher internal temperature than 111°F. The problem is *listeria* is found in foods that you don't normally heat, such as lunch meat, unpasteurized soft cheese, such as feta and brie, as well as Mexican-style soft cheeses. Pregnant women should avoid these unpasteurized soft cheeses for just this reason because there's not going to be a possibility of killing listeria if it's in these soft cheeses. So again, if you're pregnant or contemplating pregnancy, avoid soft cheeses.

Shigella oftentimes is associated with poor personal hygiene of the food handlers, and is the main cause, so just about any food can carry it. Again, these bacteria enter the intestinal tract and start to produce a toxin within the intestinal tract. But the big one here is *E. coli* in its varying strains. The CDC estimates that 70,000 people become ill each year from *E. coli* and some people are going to die from it. So where does the *E. coli* come from? It comes from fecal matter in the food or the water supply. So again, it's that inability to wash your hands in a very respectful way after using restaurant facilities.

It can contaminate undercooked meat, unpasteurized apple juice, and certainly, there have been outbreaks. Many, many of the food manufacturers are now looking at unpasteurized juices as a healthier alternative to pasteurized, but when you pasteurize a juice and you heat it to high temperatures, yes, you may kill or denature some of the beneficial compounds that are in that juice, but you're also killing the pathogenic bacteria. Raw sprouts can also be a source because raw sprouts, again, are very difficult to wash. Once the *E. coli* gets embedded into that sprouting mixture, it becomes difficult to wash it out. Since you know that you would do a better job of washing produce maybe than the food handler would, eating raw sprouts at home would be the safest bet that you can control infection. My recommendation would be to avoid that in a salad bar. Fresh produce can be contaminated as well as water, so again, *E. coli* is going to be the one that most of us see in the press and certainly, the one that most of the tainted food is going to be contaminated with.

Campylobacter jejuni can contaminate raw meat, uncooked poultry, unpasteurized milk, and untreated water. I have to tell you, in my clinical practice, I see a lot of individuals who are going out to dairy farms and buying unpasteurized milk, believing that it is more natural and is going to help their immune system rally around bacteria because they're going to be exposed to that bacteria in the unpasteurized milk. I would really dissuade individuals from doing that. Certainly, if you grew up on a farm, you might have had unpasteurized milk, but as a family strategy, always choose the pasteurized milk.

Staph and botulism are usually separate from the other diseases because they behave a little bit differently. They produce toxins, sometimes referred to as "enterotoxins," "entero" meaning gastrointestinal tract. Bacteria can grow on the food. It releases toxins and it's the toxin that causes the illness in the person consuming this toxic food. *Staph. aureus* is one of those bacteria. In almost all healthy humans, we carry this bacteria in our nose, so it's easily transmitted to food through coughing, sneezing, and improper food handling. So if you go to a salad bar, that's one of the reasons why they have a sneeze guard there, to prevent the contamination of that food.

Clostridium botulinum is a little bit different. It can occur in improperly home-canned foods. Certainly, you can see sometimes the scratch and dent sale at the grocery store, if a food is dented or it has a leaky seal or a bulge, pass it by, even though it's a good bargain because again, you certainly don't want to end up with a botulism infection by trying to save a few pennies at the grocery store. The symptoms are different than other food-borne illnesses. Food-borne illnesses usually have those gastrointestinal side effects, but with botulism, there's blurred or double vision, difficulty swallowing, speaking, or breathing. The reason is it's somewhat paralytic in nature. If someone has ever had botox injections, actually what you're doing is injecting botulism into the muscle to relax it. So it makes sense that botulism is going to cause a different sign or symptom. It's not necessarily gastrointestinal, but it may be swallowing, speaking, or breathing difficulties because you've paralyzed muscles.

More information about all these food-borne illnesses can be found at the USDA or the FDA websites listed in your guidebook. Well, what about chemical contamination of food? Generally, we don't think about this, but certainly, this can be a cause of illness. Chemical cross-contamination can be reduced by diligent washing. Now, certainly, cleaners and sanitizers are used in food production facilities or in food service preparation, and can be absorbed by the food and cross-contaminate. So keep in mind that it may be the establishment's attempt to try and keep you healthy and safe. They're cleaning down their equipment, and it's not rinsed or processed appropriately, and lo and behold, you've had a contamination from a chemical, not bacteria.

Certainly, skins of fruits and vegetables can become broken and contaminated with pesticides or other agricultural chemicals. Plant and animal toxins, agricultural chemicals, and industrial chemicals can also be part of that chemical contamination. What about physical methods? There's a concept called "physical cross-contamination," and any foreign material that doesn't belong in that product, such as glass, bone, metal, or plastic, can end up in food.

I actually had an incident where I was using medical-grade whey protein for some of my athletes, and I couldn't get the product any more. I called the manufacturer and I said, "what's the delay? Why can't I buy this whey protein?" The company told me they rejected all their base material because the whey protein was contaminated with glass shards. This would be an example of a product that was rejected because it had a foreign material. Unfortunately, if it wasn't caught at the processing, you could have been the consumer that consumed the glass shards, so again, sometimes these foreign bodies or foreign materials can be a problem. These items usually cause contamination by an accident in the production facility where the food is being processed, so certainly, finding plastic or glass in your food would be another way that you could get ill, but again, it wouldn't be bacteria.

Are there certain populations that are at risk? Well, the answer is absolutely yes. These populations are going to experience more severe symptoms, and are at higher risk for contracting a food-borne illness. Certainly, infants and very young children—this is one of the reasons why infants shouldn't be fed honey under the age of two years because there might be trace amounts of botulism. Adults are going to be sort of protected from that. Young infants and children are not. Other populations are the elderly, individuals greater than 65 years old. If, for whatever reasons, you have an immune compromised situation, such as HIV disease. Chronic illnesses, like diabetes and cancer that might alter your immune system, as well as pregnant women.

What are the consequences of food-borne illness? Well, many cases go unreported and usually the estimates of the causes of the symptoms are based on reports by health-care professionals and health departments. This is usually associated with a bacterial contamination. The usual symptoms that you would experience from a food-borne illness would include diarrhea, and this may actually be bloody diarrhea, abdominal cramping, chills, fever, vomiting, and dehydration. But would you experience any of those if the contamination was a glass shard? Maybe not.

We also have food safety regulating agencies, and as I said, the United States' food supply is one of the safest in the world. We have a safety net system here of individuals, as well as organizations, that sole method or sole source is going to be, can I protect you from a food-borne illness? The goal here of all these organizations is disease prevention, and there are many different levels involved, including federal, state, local public health agencies, as well as the private sector. The goal always here is that these agencies work as a team.

Once an illness develops, a local health agency is usually the first to respond. If indeed it looks like it's an epidemic in proportion, then state and federal levels become involved, if necessary. So if your favorite restaurant has an outbreak of food-borne illness, it may be only your local agency that responds because there's no need for state and federal levels to become involved. But at the federal level, there are three agencies that are involved, each with different duties. Certainly, the Centers for Disease Control and Prevention, the CDC, are responsible for the risk assessment of public health hazards. They give us the data on how many Americans are actually infected with food-borne illnesses, and so they give us these public health advisories.

The FDA is actually involved in the regulation of low acid canned foods, imported foods—again, if you're following the news, this is oftentimes a real challenge for regulating imported foods—pasteurized milk, and certain types of seafood. The USDA Food Safety Inspection Service, FSIS, regulates pasteurized eggs, the grading of shell eggs for quality, meat, poultry, including the slaughter and processing procedures that are used.

We also have a system called "Hazard Analysis Critical Control Point," and my guess is most of you all have not heard of that before, but it is a federal process designed to keep our food supply safe. This program was first used in the 1960s for the space program, and it provided 100% assurance against contamination. Protecting astronauts and individuals going into space was really key because dealing with a food-borne illness that far away from home was going to be difficult to manage. Since then, this system has undergone changes and modifications, and is still widely used in the United States today in dairy, seafood, juice, meat processing, and other industries, although there is no labeling for it. You can't go to the grocery store and find this labeling on the packaged food. It's one of those things behind the scenes that's going on to keep our food supply safe.

What about prevention methods? What are the agencies' roles? Certainly, food safety regulation legislation that controls processing and handling practices is very important. Some of the new things that are up and coming are about the irradiation of foods. Some believe that this would be effective in decreasing the rates of food-borne illnesses. Why might it be effective? Because it's going to destroy bacteria and other viruses present on the food. An example of prions is going to be mad cow disease. For example, prions, toxins, pesticides, and mercury are all resistant to radiation, so again, although it may destroy bacteria and viruses, there are other things in our food supply. Certainly, we all had concerns with mad cow disease. That's going to be resistant to the effects of radiation.

Foods can still become contaminated after irradiation in processing plants, grocery stores, or at home. Although the initial plan was that irradiating the food supply is going to eliminate food-borne illnesses, that can't be true because there are so many places along the supply chain where food could become contaminated. Additionally, fruits and vegetables would develop a change in flavor and texture when irradiated, and I think for most American consumers, there is a little bit of a concern with this way of protecting the food supply, so you see this less in the newspaper these days.

Now what about you? What about you as the consumer? Consumer behaviors that influence food safety are, first and foremost, we know hand-washing is a must when we prepare food for our family. According to the CDC, this is the single most important means of preventing the spread of food-borne illnesses caused by bacteria. When I first started at the Texans, our players are going from the football field to the cafeteria, with no time in between to even use the restroom, so we ended up putting instant hand sanitizing gels in our cafeteria, in the locker room, pretty much anywhere in the football facility to reduce the incidence of food-borne infections. So again, if you're traveling and you don't have access to water, think about using those instant hand sanitizing gels and carry those with you in your car.

If you're going to wash your hands, it takes about 20 seconds to sanitize your hands. So think about singing the ABCs, and quite honestly, this is a great way to teach it to your children and your grandchildren. Warm water and soap, suds up, and again, sing the ABCs. If your children don't like really hot water, and I'm going to say probably most of us don't like to have our hands under scalding water, just keep in mind it's the contact with the soap and the mechanical action of rubbing your hands that's important. You also need to scrub between fingers and underneath fingernails to make sure that you don't have some kind of food-borne activity going on underneath your fingernails or in your hands.

Dry your hands with a paper towel, not a dirty dishcloth. So again, you've spent all this time in washing and cleaning your hands, and then you dry them off on something that wasn't very clean. Certainly, keeping the temperature of the food away from the danger zone is really important, so what is the danger zone? If food is between 41°F to 135°F, that's where bacteria are going to grow the best, so store your foods at the appropriate temperature. Here's a tip for you. Thermometers rule. If you have a refrigerator, let's say it's an older refrigerator, you need to make sure that you have a refrigerator thermometer to make sure that the foods that are in your refrigerator are stored below that magical 40°F mark.

Certainly, again, keeping hot foods hot (above 135°F), as well as your cold foods cold (below 40°F) is really pretty key. Again, you can't guess. You have to have a thermometer. Never ever leave perishable foods like egg salads, meat, and dairy products at room temperature for more than two hours. Well, a lot of that depends on where you live. If I live in south Texas, I have temperatures that are 95° probably six months out of the year, so we have to modify that recommendation and never leave perishable foods at room temperature for more than an hour if the temperature is 90°.

Let's think about this for a second. You're going on a picnic and you just have to stop at Grandma's to pick something up, so you left all your food in the car. Well, now that car temperature rises. It gets to above 120°, maybe 130°, in the car, and you've now narrowed down that window of safety. Again, the key point is if in doubt, throw it out. When we're talking about keeping these things at room temperature for more than two hours, that also includes preparation, serving, and cleanup time. When you're trying to cool large amounts of food quickly, use shallow containers because, again, the quicker I cool off that food if I'm going to refrigerate leftovers, the less likely I am to have pathogenic bacteria grow.

Thawing food. Refrigeration or under cool running water are the best methods when thawing foods for preparation. Do not leave food sitting out on counters to defrost because again, the outer surface of that meat is not going to stay cool enough when the inside is still frozen. Keep in mind that includes your Thanksgiving turkey. Do not let that sit out on the counter for three or four hours and think, well, I'm going to cook it. I'm not going to use a meat thermometer. I don't think you want to be serving up food poisoning at your Thanksgiving dinner.

Cook foods to their appropriate internal temperature, and you can find a list of recommended temperatures in your guidebook. Again, if you're not sure what it needs to be, keep in mind use that thermometer and check in your guidebook. A kitchen thermometer is your best bet to, again, determine the internal temperature of food products. Another way of looking at this is that you have to have a little bit of detective work in your refrigerator. First in, first out. When you're at home, be sure to check the dates on food labels, and discard any food that is questionable. It's not just past its expiration date, but is it discolored, smells odd, or in other ways is not normal? Now, again, keep in mind that oftentimes foods that are spoiled may not necessarily have discoloration or smell odd, so again, be very diligent with your food preparation and handling.

Clean hands for everybody involved are a must, either through thorough washing or gloves. Raw meat utensils should be separated from other foods and utensils used in preparation. In my kitchen, I have my kitchen sink right in the middle, and then I always mess with my raw meats on one side of the kitchen counter, and my vegetables on the other. That way, I don't have any cross-contamination on my kitchen counter. Although it's not always possible to determine exactly where food-borne illnesses originate, recent CDC studies show of the reported cases, just over half are traced to restaurants, delis, cafeterias, and hotels, but about 18% were attributed at home, so we all have to be careful. We all have to be diligent.

What about emergency preparedness? Natural disasters can occur with little notice, and people do not realize the importance of food safety with power outages, flooding, and lack of resources to obtain food. Living in south Texas, we had the unfortunate circumstance of Hurricane Ike, and I can tell you that I did not have a generator. I was not prepared for that, and so within about two hours of my food in my refrigerator reaching room temperature, it all had to be discarded. Certainly, in areas of flooding, you can have flooded or contaminated water that can get into the food supply. When we lived in New Orleans when my husband was in medical school, my son got giardiasis, which is a parasitic poisoning from the New Orleans water supply. As the water flooded and went into the city water supply, we all had this wonderful experience with a parasitic infection.

The USDA has numerous useful emergency preparedness fact sheets on its website, and it's listed in your guidebook. These sheets cover details with emergencies before, during, and after they happen. The one thing that arises frequently is how long can the food stay in the refrigerator or the freezer without power? An unopened refrigerator in general will keep food safe for about 4 hours. A full freezer, and the key here is full, will hold the temperature for about 48 hours. If your freezer's only half-full, it's about 24 hours. So oftentimes, we describe it as food safety, it's in your hands. And I think these are all key points in keeping you safe. Always wash your hands. Respect the temperature gradient. Again, if in doubt, throw it out.

Frequently asked questions. How do I know the difference between symptoms of a food-borne illness and those of a viral intestinal disease, such as stomach flu? It's hard to determine because the symptoms are similar, so again, you may have the same consequences of diarrhea, dehydration, all of those other kinds of GI issues, but you may not be able to tell the difference. Now, certainly, if you've been at a picnic or you've eaten out at an unknown restaurant, those might be the tipoff that it's a food-borne illness and not stomach flu, but not a guarantee.

If you're like me, I spend a lot of time at my desk, what happens if you bring a frozen TV dinner-type lunch? Do you need to keep it frozen until you microwave it, or is it okay to leave it on your desk for a couple of hours? Well, I got to tell you, you either got to refrigerate it or consider using a thermometer to check the internal temperature if you insist on leaving it on the desk. I think that is a real challenge, so I actually went out and bought a small refrigerator for my office because I didn't want to chance it, and I have a little refrigerator thermometer to make sure that it's below 40°.

Another frequently asked question. "My son has allergies, so I'd like to prepare his school lunch. I can't refrigerate it though. What do I do to keep his food safe until mealtime?" It's pretty simple. Freeze your juice-pack boxes and use them as a lunchbox cold pack. If your son or daughter doesn't drink juice, you could try actually taking a bottle of water, unscrewing the top, pouring off an ounce or two, and freezing that. That way, as the water expands when it freezes, you're not going to have a cracked plastic bottle in the lunch kit. So that might be another strategy that you can use. It can keep that cold food cold because again, if it's sitting in that locker all day long, it's not going to be safe.

Another question. I've been on vacation. How can I tell if a weather emergency has occurred when I was gone? One of the things that you can do is you put an ice cube in a plastic container in the freezer. If it's melted and reformed, you'll be able to see that the freezer was off for a considerable amount of time. And again, it may be hard to discard food that you don't think is safe, but again, you don't want to be one of those 325,000 individuals that is hospitalized for a food-borne illness.

Another concern is, If we cool foods in shallow containers on the counter, and then place in the fridge, isn't it bad to put hot food right into the refrigerator? I learned this from my mother. Don't ever put hot food in the refrigerator because it's going to wear out the motor of the refrigerator. But again, I'm going to tell you common sense rules. Put those hot foods in a shallow pan and refrigerate it. You don't want to take a roast that's at 170° and directly place it into the refrigerator. Let it cool off a little bit, maybe 15, 20 minutes, but refrigerate it as soon as possible.

Children being children, another frequently asked question is "my daughter does not like to wash her hands in hot water, especially for 20 seconds." Well, back down the temperature of the water. Realize that her skin is a little bit more sensitive than maybe yours is, but make it a game. Sing the ABCs. If that's not her favorite song, find a favorite song that goes on for about 20 seconds and make it a pleasant experience. Sometimes you can get the little soaps that are scented or nicely colored to entice her. Sometimes I'll have families that actually put up a sticker chart that every time I catch you washing your hands and singing the song, I'm going to put a star on a star chart for you. After you've completed all your stars, we'll have a special trip.

Hopefully, these tips on food safety have been important, and thank you very much.

Demystifying Food Labels
Lecture 28

> A tip for you might be not to be hooked in by an ingredient on the front label. You have to flip over the back of the package and read the food label.

In May 1994, the Nutrition Labeling and Education Act made vast changes to the regulations surrounding food labeling. The aim was to encourage consumers to make more healthful food choices and to encourage food manufacturers to make more nutritionally sound food items. All food labels must now provide certain specified information.

Here are some tips for healthier consumption. Always examine the back of the package for nutrition information. Pay close attention to the serving size and the number of servings in a package. Next, check the number of calories and the calories from fat. Make sure that the calories you are consuming are not mostly from fat. Aim for less than 5% of the daily value for fat, saturated fat, cholesterol, and sodium. Aim for more than 20% for fiber, calcium, iron, vitamin A, and vitamin C.

Aim for less than 5% of the daily value for fat, saturated fat, cholesterol, and sodium.

How do you recognize a sugar on a label? Added sugars include corn syrup, high-fructose corn syrup, maltose, dextrose, honey, maple syrup, and fruit juice concentrate. Remember that the ingredients in the food are listed from the most to the least by weight.

There are FDA-approved exceptions to every rule, including nutrients on a food label. "Total calories from fat" can be deleted from the food label if the food item has less than 0.5 g of fat per serving. The label can state "0 trans fat" if there is less than 0.5 g of trans fat per serving. "Total cholesterol per serving" can be deleted if the food has less than 2 mg of cholesterol per serving and if the product makes no claims about fat, cholesterol, or fatty acids. "Total fiber per serving" can be deleted if the product contains less than a gram of fiber per serving. "Total sugars per serving" can be deleted if the food item contains less than a gram of sugar per serving and makes no claims about sugars, sweeteners, or sugar alcohol content. Grams of protein must always be listed, but the "percent daily value" can be deleted.

The FDA has established specific definitions for the terminology found in labeling and packaging. "Good source" means the food item must provide between 10% and 19% of the daily value for a given substance per serving. "Light" means the food item contains 50% or less fat than another brand or than the regular version of a food item made by the same manufacturer. "Fat free" means the food item has less than 0.5 g of fat per serving and no added oil or fat. "Low in sodium" means the food item has no more than 140 mg of sodium per serving. "High fiber" means the food item contains at least 5 g of fiber per serving.

A study showed that Americans may be making serious mistakes in food selection. Other studies confirm that food labels are useful in helping people monitor and reduce their fat intake, but they also acknowledge that there are populations that still need to be reached.

What is the future of nutrition labeling? Supermarkets may become bigger players in labeling products, which may create even more confusion for consumers. The numerous versions of labels and nutrition information can be detrimental for those with special needs. Front-of-package labeling will be trend based.

Let's review some frequently asked questions. What's the difference between "low fat" and "low calories"? "Low fat" means that the food item has less than 3 g of fat per serving. "Low calories" means that the food item has fewer than 40 calories per serving.

If I only have time to look at a couple of things on a label, what should they be? Look for portions per package, calories, and things that are important to your personal health.

Table 18. FDA food-labeling terms

Term	Meaning
	General terms
Good source	Provides 10%–19% of the daily value for a given substance per serving.
Free	This product is without (does not contain) whatever term precedes it.
Low	You can consume this item frequently without surpassing a nutrient's daily value.
Less	Contains at least 25% fewer calories from a specified nutrient than another brand or food item.
High; rich in; excellent in	Contains 20% or greater of a specified nutrient's daily value.
	Terms concerning fats
Fat-free	Has less than 0.5 g of fat per serving and has no added oil or fat.
Light	Contains 50% or less than another brand or than the "regular" version of the food item made by the same manufacturer (e.g., Kraft Mayonnaise versus Kraft Light Mayonnaise). However, with oils, "light" refers to the color.
Low-fat	Has 3 g or less of fat per serving.
Less fat	Contains 25% or less than another brand or than the regular version of the food item made by the same manufacturer.
Extra lean	Contains less than 95 mg of cholesterol, 5 g of fat, and 2 g of saturated fat per 100 g of poultry, seafood, or meat and per serving.
Lean	Contains less than 95 mg of cholesterol, 10 g of fat, and 4.5 g of saturated fat per 100 g of poultry, seafood, or meat and per serving.

| Mono- and diglycerides | Ingredients in food that are forms of fat. Fat in food is found primarily as a triglyceride. A monoglyceride is added for creaminess and is a fatty acid esterified to a glycerol backbone. |

Terms concerning fiber and sodium

High-fiber	Contains at least 5 g of fiber per serving.
Light	The item is low in calories and the manufacturer has reduced its sodium content by at least 50%.
Low in sodium	Has less than or equal to 140 mg of sodium per serving.
Very low sodium	Contains less than or equal to 35 mg of sodium per serving.
Sodium-free; salt-free	Has 5 mg or less of sodium per serving.

Terms concerning calories

Light	Has 1/3 fewer calories per serving than another food item (either from a competitor's brand or the same brand by the manufacturer).
Low-calorie	Has 40 calories or fewer per serving.
Calorie-free	Has fewer than 5 calories per serving.
Reduced-calorie	Has at least 25% fewer calories than another food item per serving (from the same or a different manufacturer).

Terms concerning cholesterol

Less cholesterol	Contains at least 25% less cholesterol compared to another food item and contains 2 g or less of saturated fat per serving.
Low-cholesterol	Has 20 mg or less of cholesterol and 2 g or less of saturated fat per serving.
Cholesterol-free	Has less than 2 mg of cholesterol and 2 g or less of saturated fat per serving.

Source: Data from U.S. Food and Drug Administration, *Guidance for Industry*.
Note: g = gram; mg = milligram. ■

Suggested Reading

Brown, A., *Understanding Food*, chap. 28.

Brown, J., *Nutrition Now*, unit 6.

Questions to Consider

1. How will you apply the suggestions for reading food labels when you shop?

2. What examples might you have of being misled by an advertisement or food claim on a particular product?

Demystifying Food Labels
Lecture 28—Transcript

Hello, and welcome back. Imagine this: You're in the grocery store, you're looking at food labels on five different cereals or five cans of soup or wholegrain breads, and which one do you choose? How do you sort out the front of the package and the back of the package? A tip for you might be not to be hooked in by an ingredient on the front label. Just because a food says "turkey" on the front, and you think, that's a lean protein, this is all good, don't be fooled and think, okay, because it says turkey, automatically that's a better food choice for me. You have to flip over the back of the package and read the food label.

We all have read a food label. We know it's required by law to include the ingredients of a particular food, such as calories, fats, protein, sodium, fiber, and other nutrients per serving. Because there's so much legislation and legalities associated with food labeling, I think oftentimes people become inundated and think, well, I'm just going to choose by the ingredients and not necessarily look at that nutrition facts panel. But what do we really need to know to read a food label that can help us to make wise choices? Because that's the point, isn't it? We want to use the nutrition labeling on a food to make a better or more helpful choice, or in reverse, avoid a food ingredient that we may have a sensitivity to.

Here are some useful tips for healthier consumption, what to look for in the grocery store. First and foremost, always examine the back of the package for nutrition information. A key consideration here is, does is list what you're going to purchase as a food? Your tip is going to be it will have a nutrition facts panel, or is it actually a supplement, and the label on the back of the package is going to say, "supplement facts panel"? So again, we have two abilities to buy a whey protein product. One, you flip it over and it has nutrition facts panel, and the other product has a supplement facts panel. You must know that a nutrition facts panel or a food is going to be regulated in a different way than a supplement.

When you're looking at this label and you've actually decided what you're purchasing is a food with a nutrition facts panel, pay very close attention to the serving size and the number of servings in a package. I'll give you a great example. I was looking at diabetic candy bars, and I looked at the label. Just like you, I screened it very quickly, and I saw that per serving, it had 70 calories, and I thought, wow, a candy bar at 70 calories. Actually, when I looked at the number of servings, it had seven in the candy bar. So the reality was it wasn't such a good deal. In fact, it had more calories than the regular version at about twice the cost. Before you buy the food, you have to be realistic with yourself on how many servings you are likely to eat in a sitting.

Here's another example. The nutrition label on a personal pepperoni pizza says something like 210 calories, 70 calories from fat, 8 grams of fat, 3.5 grams of saturated fat, 520 milligrams of sodium, and automatically that doesn't make it sound delicious, does it? But it doesn't sound all that bad. But then you look at the serving information, and that's for one-fourth of the pizza. Although the front of the package said "personal pan pizza," it's not so personal because how likely is it that you're only going to eat a fourth of that tiny little pizza and call it a meal? Well, the whole personal pan pizza will have 840 calories, 280 coming from fat, 32 grams of total fat, and 14 grams are saturated. Almost an entire day's allowance for sodium at 2080 milligrams. Keep in mind that the USDA recommends sodium being no more than 2300 milligrams per day, so you've now almost reached your maximum in one item at one meal.

Next, check the number of calories and the calories from fat. The FDA gives a general guideline to calories per serving that states if it's less than 40 calories, it can be considered or labeled "low." A hundred calories is moderate, and 400 calories or more are high. Now, I want you to think about how many times you've gone to the grocery store and actually seen something that's labeled a "high calorie source." That probably wouldn't be a big seller at the grocery store. Not as many people are trying to gain weight as lose weight. So I think, again, even though there are requirements in terms of how you can say something, it doesn't mandate that all this information is on the package.

Also, look to make sure that the calories that you are consuming are not mostly from fat. Keep in mind that the more processed the food becomes, the more likely it is to have trans fat. The more shelf-stable a food becomes, the more likely it is to have saturated fat that's a little bit more shelf-stable than a polyunsaturated fat would be. So keep in mind that you want to make sure that you're not getting all your calories in that product from fat. You also want to make sure that you're limiting your fat, sodium, and cholesterol intake. Keep in mind that not everybody is going to have the same health concerns. So if cholesterol is up at the top of your list, you might want to quickly flip that over and say, okay, I want to choose a food based on its cholesterol content. Limiting your intake of these nutrients as a prevention model lowers your risk of obesity, heart disease, and other disease states that we'll get into later.

Be aware when you're reading that label that foods that have a higher sodium content may not always taste salty. Oftentimes, people think, well, I can't have that bag of chips because I can taste the salt. That must be absolutely unbelievably high in sodium. You flip over the back of the package and it's got 150 milligrams of sodium. Now you look at your breakfast cereal. It doesn't taste salty, but it's got 590 milligrams of sodium. Don't be confused by the taste alone. Baked goods, cereals, cheeses, prepared foods, and even candy can contain more salt or sodium than you might expect. Again, that's the beauty of that nutrition facts panel.

Another guideline is to get enough fiber, vitamin A, vitamin C, calcium, and iron. Eating enough of these nutrients can lower your risk of certain disease states. But also if your iron in your blood is elevated, and it's usually men that have elevated levels of iron, you can avoid iron-fortified foods by looking at the back of that package label. So again, you don't want to choose a breakfast cereal that says 100% of the daily value for iron if you know that you've got too much iron in your blood.

Be familiar on the back of that package with what's called "percent daily values." Keep in mind this is based on a 2000 calorie diet, so it might be more or less for you, depending on how many calories you require in a day. Roughly 5% of the daily value of a particular nutrient is low, and 20% of the daily value is considered high. Aim for less than 5% of the daily value for fat, saturated fat, cholesterol, and sodium. Aim for more of the good stuff. Aim for more than 20% for fiber, calcium, iron, vitamin A, and vitamin C. So what you're trying to do is use that nutrition facts panel to stay away from the stuff you want to get rid off, and maximize those that you want a little bit more of. Also make sure to account for these numbers when you're accounting for the number of servings in the package or your individual serving size.

One of my favorite things to look for on a label is sugars, and how do recognize a sugar on a label? If you're concerned with the amount of sugar you're consuming, be sure to look on the ingredient list to verify there are no added sugars. That's a key take-home point. You're now looking at the ingredient list for added sugars. Some commonly added sugars include corn syrup, high-fructose corn syrup, and some you may not be familiar are maltose, dextrose, honey, maple syrup, and fruit juice concentrate. All of those are going to be sources of added sugar from the manufacturer. Keep in mind if you're looking at an ingredient list, sugar ends in "ose." Now, again, certainly, maple syrup, fruit juice concentrate, are not going to have "ose" in them, but maltose, dextrose, sucrose will all have "ose." That is the tip for looking for sugar on the label.

However, it's a little muddy here because in an eight-ounce glass of milk, there are 12 grams of sugar on that nutrition facts panel. So you're looking at a glass of milk and you think, okay, the manufacturer must have added sugar to this product. No, this is something that Mother Nature put in that product. The carbohydrate that is in milk is lactose, and lactose is a disaccharide, two sugar units stuck together, so the 12 grams of sugar in milk are coming from lactose. Yes, it is a sugar, but not added by the manufacturer. So again, you go to your ingredient list, and for milk on the ingredient list, you might see milk, vitamin A, and vitamin D, but you don't see any high-fructose corn syrup. You don't see any maltose or dextrose. So you know that the sugar that was in there was natural.

The same thing if you're getting unsweetened applesauce. It's going to tell you it might have 15 grams of sugar, but you look at the ingredient list, and there's no added sugar. So again, keep in mind that the nutrition facts panel is not necessarily going to identify where the sugar came from on the label, but it's going to be in the ingredient list. To limit nutrients that have no more than a percent daily value, like trans fats and sugars—in other words, there's no value needed, there's no amount of this that's required—look at the labels and choose the food with the lowest amount to minimize your intake. Remember that the list of all ingredients of the food is listed from the most to the least, and this is done by weight. So again, if you're wondering if there's a lot of trans fat in this food, and you look at the ingredient list, and lo and behold, your first ingredient is hydrogenated vegetable oil—hydrogenated means, essentially, a trans fat, partially hydrogenated means a trans fat— if that's first on your ingredient list, that would be a product that you want to avoid.

Another tip when you're looking at this ingredient list is the more ingredients in the food product, in general, the more processed the food, particularly if you don't understand the ingredients. So if you have to have a degree in biochemistry to understand what's in your food, and there are words you've never heard of before, you can generally assume that the more ingredients, or the less you understand that label, the more processed the food becomes. Again, keep in mind that we're trying to stay away from processed foods and eat more whole foods.

Don't be fooled. There are FDA approved exceptions to every rule, including nutrients on a food label. Total calories from fat can be deleted from the food label. It doesn't have to be there if the food item has less than 0.5 grams of fat per serving. Again, be really careful about the portion size because a way that a manufacturer can get around this, remember that diet candy bar? What they've done is take a candy bar that most of us would consider a single serving and they've now dissected it into seven. So they don't have to put that on the label because the portion size is so small, each portion is going to have less than 0.5 grams of fat per serving.

Likewise, a company may still be able to claim 0 trans fat if there's less than 0.5 grams of trans fat per serving in their product. The key here is serving, so again, if they're trying to minimize the negative publicity of trans fats on their label, they just make the portion sizes smaller and then again, they are in compliance with the legislation. So keep in mind that even though there may be a law associated with it, the manufacturer is in charge of the portion sizes. In compliance with this rule, manufacturers can reduce their portion size to have 0 grams of trans fat, so that's the key take-home message.

As consumers focus on trans fats, manufacturers have switched from trans fat back to saturated fat to meet the consumer's perception of heart healthy. Keep in mind that a lot of this is the difference between the front of the package and the back of the package. The front of the package is going to be designed to market to you. The back of the package, where the facts label is, has to be in compliance with the law, although there are ways of skirting that a little bit.

Certainly, total cholesterol per serving may also be deleted from the food label if the food has less than 2 milligrams of cholesterol per serving, and if that product makes no claims about fat, cholesterol, or fatty acids. Companies may also delete total fiber per serving from their label if indeed their product contains less than a gram of fiber per serving. It's kind of like don't ask, don't tell. Basically, they're not giving you the information that their product is a poor source of fiber. They're just giving you no information.

A company may also delete total sugars per serving from the product label if the food item contains less than a gram of sugar per serving, and make no claims about sugars, sweeteners, or sugar alcohol content. Sugar alcohols are in foods to reduce the sugar, but again, you can look at that word and say, "if it ends in "ol," such as sorbitol, manitol, xylitol, or lactilol, any of these "ol" words is going to be a sugar alcohol." Make sure you look at that ingredient list.

A company must always list the grams of protein that product contains, but the percent daily value may be deleted from the label. It can be deleted if the protein claim is not made, or if the food item is for infants or children less than four years old. The reason is they require less protein, and again, protein is a little bit difficult to navigate because it depends on how much protein for growth and development, your ideal body weight, etc.

Terminology found in labeling and packaging. We've seen food-related items like "light," "low fat," "high fiber" on packaging and labels, but do you know what they really mean? The FDA has established specific definitions for these terms. We can't review all of them, but I'm going to give you a few, and the rest are going to be listed in your guidebook. So it's almost like you have to have a degree in law, oftentimes, to make sure that you can navigate a food label. So if indeed it is called a "good source," and that's a "front of packaging" word, it means this food item must provide between 10% and 19% of the daily value for a given substance per serving. The word "light" means that the food item contains 50% or less fat than another brand, or of the regular version of a food item if it's made by the same manufacturer.

An exception to that would be, say, for example, olive oil. Olive oil that's labeled "light" oftentimes means light in color, not light in calories. So we get so used to seeing light that we think "light" means less calories, light beer, and so on. We can come up with a lot of different examples. But "light" when it comes to oil really means light in color. "Fat free" means that the food item has to have less than 0.5 grams of fat per serving, and has no added oil or fat in the food. "Low in sodium" means that the food item has less than or equal to 140 milligrams of sodium per serving. So I want you to think about this the next time you go to the grocery store and you're buying a sports drink. Most of the sports drinks on the shelf today have 110 milligrams of sodium per serving, and they could legitimately market themselves as low in sodium. They don't do that because they're trying to market themselves as replacing the electrolytes lost in sweat, but actually, it meets the definition of a lower sodium food.

"High fiber" means that the food item contains at least 5 grams of fiber per serving, and again, you might want to take your guidebook along the next time you go grocery shopping to be able to navigate the legislative words that are going to be on your packaging. So does this stuff actually work? What does the research say about the American diet and food labels? Are we actually taking all this government-sponsored legislation and translating this into making better food choices? Well, a study by Hrovat and colleagues at the University of Cincinnati asked 200 men and women to choose between two fabricated cookie packages. These were not real cookies. On the front label, one said "Low fat" and the other said "No saturated fat." And 84% of participants made their product choice without looking at the nutrition label on the back of packages.

What does that mean? Keep in mind that when you're buying something off a grocery store shelf, you're drawn to that product by the front of the package, not necessarily the back. So if there are key buzz words that appeal

153

to you, you're much more likely to choose a product based on the front of the package versus the back. Furthermore, in this study, 64% of participants chose the "no saturated fat" label over the "low fat" package label. That's not a bad idea, but the consumer might actually miss the total calories by not reading the label. In my family, we have a lot of bad history of heart disease, and so I've actually taught my children that it's not necessarily the total fat that they want to look for, but it's the saturated fat. Again, your family may actually have some key things that you want to look for on the label, and that may be what you focus in on.

What is the implication of this particular study? Americans may be making serious mistakes in food selection, and consequently, their overall health, by not reading and closely inspecting nutrition labels on the back of food items. The results of other studies confirm that food labels are useful in helping people monitor and reduce their fat intake, but they also acknowledge that populations of persons who still need to be reached, such as seniors, men, and people who have less formal education. Also, I want you to think about this for a second. How big is that label on the back of the package? If I forget my glasses at home, I may not actually be able to read the nutrition facts panel, but I might again be attracted to that front-of-package labeling.

What is the future of nutrition labeling? Supermarkets may become a bigger player in labeling products on their shelves in their grocery store. This should make sense because the supermarket, particularly the supermarket brand, is going to be able to put whatever message they want. And the unfortunate thing is that I can go to a variety of different grocery stores, and the labeling on the store brand could be completely different, and the words on that front-label packaging may mean something completely different. Supermarket chains are creating their own labels to help identify products that are healthier, according to their own definitions. So we could go to six or seven grocery store chains and ask them for the definition of "healthy," and they may all give us a different definition.

These symbols and scores are being added to shelf tags beneath the food products, in addition to the claims that are already provided by the food label by the manufacturer. It's also on the front of the packaging. What would attract you? Now, I'll give you a great example. A major grocery store chain knows that people don't necessarily look at the back of the package for 100% whole wheat bread, so they've put caramel coloring to make the bread brown, packaged it in kind of an orange label to make the bread look browner. So they know consumers are going to pick a brown bread versus a white bread, but basically this is white bread with caramel coloring. The packaging and the messaging on the front has no true identity, no true standard.

Will this create even more confusion for consumers when they're making a purchase? I'm going to say perhaps. Each of these nutrient profiling systems uses different standards to evaluate food products. A product may receive a higher score in one store, and a lower score in another. You're scratching your head and saying, okay, if I shop at grocery store A and I buy this product, how can it not be as good for me if I'm shopping at grocery store B? So there's been almost a national movement to try and get grocery stores and other organizations to standardize that front-of-packaging labeling, and to this point, to no avail.

The graphic or the symbol is usually placed on the front of the food package, but research has yet to indicate that these symbols are registering with consumers. So do consumers know what that means? The answer at this point is no. So why are supermarkets doing this? Well, for many reasons, but they want to drive their consumers to a store brand. Now, interestingly, according to the ADA, the American Dietetic Association's Nutrition and You: Trends 2008 public opinion survey, 35% of consumers listed food package labels as credible sources of information. Now, we could look at that one or two ways. At least over a third of Americans are looking at the label. The bad news is that means 65% don't look at food label packaging as credible sources of nutrition information, despite the fact that the nutrition facts panel has legal definitions for labeling.

Fewer than 10% identified food manufacturers as credible sources. So if I'm going to interpret this for you, what this means is that at least consumers are thinking, "well, maybe manufacturers have an ulterior motive. Maybe that front-of-label packaging may not be the most credible source because it's coming from a manufacturer." According to *Nutrition Today*, consumers have also been found to trust a specific nutrition-related statement versus a general statement. For example, a statement such as "calcium-rich foods, such as skimmed milk, may reduce the risk of osteoporosis." They may believe that more than a general statement on a carton saying, for example, "good source of calcium."

The American consumer is looking for a little bit more information. Why is a good source of calcium important for me? Why must I look for a good source of calcium? Well, now, what they're doing is making a link. The legal wording associated with this is really pretty critical, though. They can't say, "skimmed milk is a good source of calcium and it will prevent osteoporosis." They can't make a prevention claim, but they may say, "reduce the risk of developing osteoporosis." There is much controversy over whether or not the current labeling of products really are giving a benefit to consumers, or to the manufacturer. Not only are the numerous labels and nutrition information overwhelming for consumers, but what about consumers who really have a unique special dietary need?

This labeling system can actually be detrimental for those who have a lactose intolerance because remember, the label is going to identify milk as having 12 grams of sugar, but not necessarily the source of that sugar. The labeling may be detrimental to individuals, say for example, with type 2 diabetes, whose primary goal is to control calories, but they're only looking for sugars on the label. What if you have celiac disease? Individuals who have celiac disease need to eliminate wheat and, probably more importantly, eliminate sources of gluten. So where wheat might be listed on the ingredient list, gluten is not. The challenge is if you have celiac disease, the nutrition facts panel, as it's currently formulated, may not give you enough information.

Certainly, high blood pressure, renal disease, all of those, again, individuals with unique nutritional concerns really are going to struggle. A person with celiac disease goes to the grocery store. They know they have to avoid wheat and gluten, but they see a label with a heart healthy symbol, and now they think, okay, if this is a healthy food, maybe it's healthy for me. And that's not going to be true. It could be a whole wheat bread or another food that's got gluten in it, and just because it has a healthy symbol on it doesn't mean it's specifically designed for people who have a gluten sensitivity.

Some of the front-of-package labeling now is listing "gluten free" wheat bread, or "gluten free" breakfast cereal, and so it's giving the consumer a little bit more information on the front of the packaging. But also keep in mind that there's no legal identity for that front-of-package labeling. I'm Joe manufacturer. I can say it's "gluten free," but I don't necessarily need to prove it's gluten free. Individuals may think the product might be healthy and they purchase it, without knowing the side effects it could produce.

Think about this from a labeling dilemma, though. Can the federal government actually give a warning on every single food product out there? I don't really think that's terribly practical. So I think the challenge is how do we provide consumers with the best information? Certainly, we can go and think about our diabetic patients who have many restrictions and guidelines as it is. With the growing population of diabetic children, this new labeling system might be even more confusing and troublesome when trying to make a healthier choice for children at such a young age. Keep in mind that if it's type 2 diabetes, the most important thing on that label is to look for total calories and calories per serving.

Just because the label says it's "low fat," however, doesn't mean that it's low in carbohydrates and sugar. So "low fat" doesn't mean it's low calorie. It just means it's reduced one segment, and we can certainly all remember the low fat craze of the 1980s and '90s, where everybody was eating low-fat cookies and low-fat candy, and we watched our American waistline grow because we never thought about calorie control.

Will the product labels actually become cluttered and overwhelming? Well, the overall goal is to reduce confusion and make it easier for consumers to buy a healthy product. But there's not one healthy product on the market that meets all of the criteria for everyone. So what do we do as consumers? Do we throw up our hands and say, "I can't navigate all the legal mumbo jumbo on a label"? If that's you, then I'm going to suggest what we do is just stick to teaching the basics. What are the basics when you go to the grocery store?

First and foremost, I always tell people to shop the perimeter. The outside aisles are where most of the best choices or the least processed foods are. Fresh produce, lean meats, low-fat dairy, and we can also throw olive oil in here, because when you look at olive oil and you flip over the back of the label, there's one ingredient. So again, we're looking for the perimeter of the store or single or maybe two-ingredient foods. We're not looking for a list of ingredients that we can't understand. Do we forget the numerous labels that have the potential to confuse many consumers in the long run? Well, maybe we do. Maybe that's just too overwhelming for you.

What about research and labeling? Will this new trend with all of this information on the package for us, will this help American consumers, or is it just another phase in the nutrition world that's going to come and go like a popular diet that people follow for a month or so, and quit in a matter of time? We'll see, but keep in mind that front-of-package labeling will be trend-based, so whatever the nutrition buzz word of the day is, low trans fat, low sugar, low carb, that's what's going to be brought to you as a consumer because it's on the front of the package. You're savvy enough to think, okay, they're marketing to me, so maybe what I want to do is flip to the back.

We're thinking about frequently asked questions. What's the difference between "low fat" and "low in calories"? First, I'm going to send you back to the guidebook. "Low fat" means that the food item has less than 3 grams of fat per serving. "Low calorie" means that the food item has less than 40 calories per serving. So if I'm a manufacturer wanting to use the "low fat" claim, but I still want my product to taste good, I might add more sugar to it to make it a little bit more palatable.

Are there labels for fresh foods, such as fruits and vegetables and meats? The answer is not necessarily. Some of the meats that are making a claim, such as a claim for a low-fat hamburger, for example, 96% fat free, lo and behold, I'm going to have to provide some nutrition information to back that up.

Another question that I get all the time is, "Reading food labels, Roberta, will add hours to my shopping time. How can I avoid that? If I've only got time to look at a couple of things on a label, what should they be?" Well, I would summarize it for you by saying portions per package, calories, and then look at things that might be individually important to you and your own personal health. Maybe in your family, it's sodium. In my family, it's saturated fat, and even trans fat. I'm going to look at those things, particularly when

I'm looking at a new product that I want to introduce to my family. Maybe you have irritable bowel and you're looking for higher fiber foods. Choose the labels and look at the back of the package to pick out things that are personally important to you, and that way, you can navigate the wonderful and oftentimes confusing world of food labels.

Thank you.

Facts on Functional Foods
Lecture 29

Many consumers believe that food is medicine, and as a dietician, I believe it can be, to a certain extent. Foods are designed to nourish us and part of that nourishment should be wellness-focused.

There has been growing concern over the research behind functional foods, and questions have been raised as to whether they really are "superfoods." Many consumers believe that food is medicine, and to a certain extent, it can be. However, we must be educated on which foods are really worth the extra punch they seem to be packing.

Let's explore functional foods. Foods are designed to nourish us, and part of that nourishment should be wellness focused. This lecture explores the definition of functional foods, gives examples of popular functional foods, explores terms used in functional food markets, and takes a look at regulations and policies regarding functional foods.

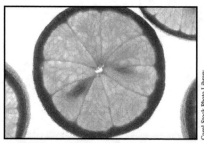

One study showed a 28% reduction in the risk of stomach cancer with a high intake of citrus fruits.

There is no legal definition of the term "functional food" in the United States. According to the American Dietetic Association, a functional food is a food that moves beyond the necessity to provide additional health benefits that may reduce disease risk or promote optimal health. Functional food categories include conventional foods, modified foods, medical foods, and foods for special dietary use.

Let's start with conventional foods. Oxygen radical absorbance capability (ORAC) is a system that gives a number to a food based on its ability to scavenge free radicals and neutralize them. Spices score high on ORAC rating tables, but the amount that you usually consume is so small that it adds little to your antioxidant intake.

All fruits, vegetables, and nuts confer antioxidant capability. These include cruciferous vegetables, tomatoes, and citrus fruit. The category of conventional foods also includes fermented dairy products, such as yogurt, which use probiotics to ferment. Another conventional food is cranberry juice, which has proanthocyanidins that reduce the risk of a urinary tract infection.

Another category is modified foods. These are modified through fortification, enrichment, or enhancement. Examples include calcium-fortified orange juice; folate-enriched bread; margarines enhanced with plant stanols or sterol esters; and energy drinks that include ginseng, guarana, or taurine. The challenge is that bioavailability information should be provided to educate the consumer on the actual amounts of the nutrient they are receiving.

Evidence-based science is emerging that links diet to chronic disease reduction and other health outcomes.

Other categories are medical foods and foods for special dietary use. medical foods have been defined by the Orphan Drug Act. A type of medical food is oral supplements designed for specific medical purposes. Foods for special dietary use do not require medical supervision. Examples of foods for special dietary use include infant foods, gluten-free foods, lactose-free foods, and foods for reduced weight.

Some 85% of consumers believe that certain foods may have health benefits that reduce the risk of chronic disease or other health concerns. Evidence-based science is emerging that links diet to chronic disease reduction and other health outcomes. There is a striving for a personalized approach to nutrition, and the wave of the future is food for the treatment of health conditions.

Is there regulation of functional foods? There is no specific regulatory framework for functional foods yet, because the movement is so new.

Currently, however, there are 3 claim categories that can be used: nutrient content claims, structure/function claims, and health claims. Establishing a cause and effect relationship with functional foods is controversial, because many factors influence food behaviors and mechanisms in the body. It is the job of the FDA and nutrition professionals to ensure that the consumer is provided with correct information.

Let's review some frequently asked questions. As a health-care professional and a mother, do you buy foods with functionality in mind? I tend to look at the whole food and not an individual ingredient.

How do I integrate functional foods into my family's diet? Choose fruits and vegetables from the colors of the rainbow; you can also look at margarines and cereals that have functional ingredients added.

Do I really have to eat mounds of healthy foods to acquire all the nutritional benefits? No, you should still watch your calorie intake. If you eat well, over time you will get enough of these wonderful nutrients in your food.

Should you go out and buy those really expensive exotic berry juices? You may want to save your money and stick to a greater whole food approach. ∎

Suggested Reading

Eskin and Tamir, *Dictionary of Nutraceuticals and Functional Foods*.

Heasman and Mellentin, *The Functional Foods Revolution*.

Questions to Consider

1. What types of functional foods do you and your family incorporate into your diet?

2. Why is FDA regulation of food claims so important to the American consumer?

Facts on Functional Foods
Lecture 29—Transcript

Greetings, and welcome back. You've been in the grocery store recently, and you've noticed exotic berry juices being exploded into the American food supply. Foods such as mangosteen, acai, and goji berry have caught the attention of the American consumer. Well, are these functional foods worth the extra money, or would any dark blue or purple juice be just as good for less money? We're going to explore that a little bit in this lecture on functional foods.

Many consumers believe that food is medicine, and as a dietician, I believe it can be, to a certain extent. Foods are designed to nourish us and part of that nourishment should be wellness-focused. However, consumers must be educated on what foods are really worth the extra punch that they seem to be packing, and foods that you might have heard of, these foods are called "functional foods." In the beginning, functional foods were thought of as preventing deficiency diseases, yet today, functional foods have taken on a whole new meaning. This lecture is going to explore the definition of functional foods, give you some examples of popular functional foods, explore some of the terms used in functional food marketing, and then take a look at the regulations and policies regarding functional foods.

Let's start out with a definition. You have to know that there's no legal definition of the term "functional food" in the United States, so there's no governmental regulations saying a functional food must be defined this way. It's rather more of a marketing strategy than it is a regulation. Well, my professional organization, the American Dietetic Association, has a definition, and a "functional food" is a food that moves beyond necessity to provide additional health benefits that may reduce disease risk or promote optimal health.

We've got some functional food categories to explore. There are going to be foods that are conventional, foods that have been modified by the manufacturer so that a functional ingredient is added in, there are medical foods that would fall into this functional food category, and foods for special dietary use. So let's start out with a whole food approach. Let's take a look at conventional foods that are unmodified.

Research has shown that fruits and vegetables were the top functional foods identified by consumers. In part, this is because fruits and vegetables have compounds and pigments with a high antioxidant capability. Now, there is a scoring or a ranking system called "ORAC" that gives a number to a food, based on its ability to scavenge free radicals. Keep in mind that what we're looking at here as we talk a lot about antioxidants, their job is to scavenge, or attack, these free radicals and neutralize them. "ORAC" stands for "oxygen radical absorbance capability," so it's given that term ORAC. Again, you can do a Google search on the Internet and you can find ORAC ratings for food.

When we look at the ORAC rating tables, spices score high on this rating, but I want you to think about this. The amount that you use is so small that it adds little to the antioxidant intake. So again, it's not that they're not powerhouses in terms of the ORAC rating, but you just don't use enough. But given typical servings, my favorite food such as dark chocolate, apples, and pomegranate juice all add relatively more to the antioxidant intake. But all fruits, vegetables, and nuts confer antioxidant capability, so I want you to think about this. You're going to the grocery store and you're thinking, should I spend the significantly higher premium on an exotic juice, or could I get something else that has a similar ORAC score? So I would encourage you to look at the ORAC scores of foods if you're going to spend a significant amount of money.

We can now take a look at examples of real foods with functional benefits. Cruciferous vegetables, such as kale and broccoli, are part of the reason why plant-focused diets are needed for cancer prevention. Naturally, they contain foods that have a significant functionality to them, and there is reduced risk of several types of cancer. It protects against carcinogenesis on experimental animals and has been shown effective in the management or prevention of stomach cancer, cancers of the esophagus, mammary glands, or breast cancer, skin, and lung. There are numerous studies pointing to the need for increasing all fruits and vegetables. So again, a key point for consumers is not to follow the new functional food of the day because I will tell you, next year it's going to be a different fruit or vegetable. Always think more fruits and vegetables. All fruits and vegetables are going to have a relatively high ORAC score, and I might want to include all of those.

Is there another group? Well, let's take a look at tomato products. Lycopene, which is part of that red pigment in tomatoes, has mixed effects in reducing certain cancers. As I mentioned before, large epidemiological studies show a relationship between low levels of lycopene in the blood and prostate cancer, but studies have not demonstrated the prevention of prostate cancer with lycopene. The FDA looked at this and found little evidence to support an association between tomato consumption and the reduced risks of prostate, ovarian, gastric, and pancreatic cancers. However, study results are still positive enough. There is an association that's developing, not necessarily cause and effect, but an association developing that's enough to say, "increase your intake of tomato products."

What about citrus fruit? Citrus fruit may reduce the risk of stomach cancer, and again, there are functional ingredients in citrus fruit that confer that benefit. One study showed a 28% reduction in the risk of stomach cancer was associated with a high intake of citrus fruits. Pooled results from observational studies show a protective effect of high citrus fruit intake and the risk of stomach cancer. So again, if you don't incorporate citrus fruit into your diet, it now might be a good idea to do so. Things like oranges would be a great example of a citrus fruit.

Certainly, in this functional category are fermented dairy products. Yogurt and other fermented food products have been shown to improve the symptoms of irritable bowel syndrome. Studies show that the short-term effects of IBS may be improved through the use of antibiotics, and then using probiotics for symptoms. Probiotics are a great example of a functional food, and again, in our conventional food category, they are there naturally to ferment the yogurt. However, there's caution here. The addition of probiotics to foods where they do not naturally occur may reduce their effectiveness. If you go to the grocery store and you hear all about probiotics, and you know that it occurs in yogurt naturally, but now you see probiotics being added to a dry food, like a cereal, you have to ask the question, when I've removed it from its parent compound and dumped it into a different food where it doesn't occur, is it going to have the same effectiveness? Again, I think that's a consideration as we look at this functional food category.

Generally speaking, if IBS can be caused by bacterial overgrowth, then killing the bad guys with an antibiotic and then turn around and replacing them with the good guys, a probiotic, may be an effective strategy. More studies are always going to be needed to prove these results for digestive conditions in the future. But again, if you're looking for a great source of a natural probiotic, think fermented foods.

Another food that gets a lot of press as a functional food is cranberry juice. Again, I'm going to caution you that taking the active ingredient in cranberry juice, which we'll explore in a second, and dehydrating it and putting it into a pill may not have the same kind of beneficial effects. So there's a lot of dried fruit and vegetable products that are on the market that you can mix in with food, but remember, there may be a change in the functionality of that ingredient when I change its form. Certainly, we've read and heard that cranberry juice can reduce the amount of bacteria in your urine, and so how does this work? What is the active ingredient? The proanthocyanidins or the dark red pigments in cranberries have been shown to inhibit the docking, or the binding, of bacteria in tissues *in vitro*, in a test tube. So basically, what it does is it prevents bacteria from binding and proliferating in the bladder, and reducing the risk of a urinary tract infection.

The use of cranberry juice and extracts as an agent against recurrent urinary tract infections is well documented in women. So if you are someone that is prone to urinary tract infections, this food may be a valuable adjunct to your diet. Now, again, keep in mind that cranberry juice is a pretty high calorie source. So indeed, if you're trying to do two things at the same time, you're trying to prevent urinary tract infections and control your weight, look for a reduced sugar version, where you're still getting the wonderful red pigments, but you reduce some of the sugar.

We have another category of functional foods called "modified foods." These are those that are modified through fortification, enrichment, or enhancement. They've taken a conventional food and they've added something with, again, that functional food enhancement to the food to improve its overall nutritional value. Let's look at some examples. Calcium-fortified orange juice is a great example. They've taken a food where calcium doesn't normally reside, orange juice, and because it's a popular breakfast item, they've added calcium to it. Again, that's a great example of a modified food that's been, again, enriched with some additional calcium. You can also see vitamin D being added to orange juice as well.

Folate-enriched bread is another example. Part of that is mandatory by the federal government, but manufacturers can add more folate to breads and again, increase their nutritional value. One of my favorite ones in this category are actually margarines that have been enhanced with plant stanols or sterol esters. What these actually do is they prevent the absorption of cholesterol from your gut. These stanols or sterol esters bind to the cholesterol receptors in your gut and prevent the cholesterol from being absorbed. This is a really nice example of taking an ingredient, a stanol or sterol ester, putting it in a margarine, and now again, reducing cholesterol.

There are certainly beverages out there with ingredients to promote energy, and we've all seen the energy drinks on the market. Things like ginseng or guarana, and guarana actually is a caffeine source. Or they might add taurine, which is an amino acid. They're taking these compounds and actually just enriching or adding an ingredient to provide additional energy.

What do we know about the research on calcium-fortified orange juice? We're going to explore this in a little bit more detail. The bioavailability of calcium from different fortification methods was tested in calcium-fortified orange juice. Results indicate that the calcium content on the labels doesn't necessarily indicate the amount of calcium that's absorbed, and this is a problem with most minerals. Just because it's on a nutrition facts panel or just because it's in a nutrition database on your computer doesn't mean that's exactly how much you absorb. So the challenge is the conclusion of this study is the information on bioavailability of fortified products should be provided to educate the consumer on the actual amounts of the nutrient they're receiving.

Controversial topics regarding functional foods include those that are genetically modified. This is using biotechnology to modify the food to improve the nutritional value, and hopefully the health. So let me give you a couple of examples. The first comes from tomatoes. There was a type of tomato called "FlavrSavr," and this was one of the first genetically modified foods introduced into the American food supply in 1994. The purpose of this genetically modified food was to improve the flavor, the shelf life, and to even reduce spoilage. So this is an example where the food was modified, so again, consumers would enjoy the flavor or the tomatoes would last a little bit longer, either at the grocery store or in the refrigerator.

Keep in mind as we start talking about these genetically modified foods that we have embraced genetically engineered hormones, such as insulin and growth hormone. Certainly, when insulin was first discovered, there are two amino acids different in pork insulin than human insulin, and so we've now gone in and genetically modified insulin to make it bioidentical to human insulin. Some of the consequences of pork insulin obviously have been eliminated. For those who have diabetes and must take insulin, this was a real boon. But when it comes to food, consumers are skeptical and have not embraced genetically modified foods. In terms of the FlavrSavr, the product is no longer available for sale.

As we think more globally about nutrition, Golden Rice is a great example of taking a look at worldwide poverty and worldwide malnutrition and genetically modifying a food. Golden Rice is a rice that's modified to contain higher amounts of beta-carotene, that precursor to vitamin A, to implement in developing countries where vitamin A deficiency is a problem. Vitamin A deficiency is one of the leading causes of childhood blindness worldwide, so adding beta-carotene to a non-perishable food is one of the best outcomes of genetically modified foods. Again, if you think about it, beta-carotene is going to come naturally from carrots and cantaloupe and anything that's going to be orange in pigment. Well, these are perishable foods, and so in regions of the world where starvation is prevalent, we can't airlift in perishable foods. Golden Rice is a great example of a genetically modified food. It is used by relief organizations now in developing countries, and again, it can contribute to the eradication of vitamin A blindness.

Another category that we're looking at is medical foods. Now, "medical foods" do have a definition, and they're defined by the Orphan Drug

Act. Medical foods are a food which is formulated to be consumed or administered enterally. Now, technically, "enterally" means by mouth, but in this case, it's really implying tube feeding. Under the supervision of a physician, and which is intended for the specific dietary management of a disease or a condition that has distinctive nutritional requirements. This is going to be based on recognized scientific principles, and are established by medical evaluation. So again, that's a long legal definition and basically, what it's saying is that they've modified a natural food to provide unique nutritional balance for someone who may have a disease with different nutritional requirements. So examples might be oral supplements that are designed for specific medical purposes, such as increased need for arginine in wound healing, or preventing muscle breakdown in cancer.

We also have a category called "foods for special dietary use," and they really don't require any medical supervision. This is a particular use for a food that's purported or represented to be used, things such as infant foods would be a great example of foods for special dietary use, gluten-free foods, foods for special dietary use, lactose-free, and foods that are being offered for reduced weight. Again, these are foods that don't have to be used under medical supervision.

Let's focus on consumers now. What do consumers believe? Well, 85% of consumers believe that certain foods may have health benefits that are going to reduce the risk of chronic disease or other health concerns. It's that belief that food is medicine, just like Hippocrates taught us centuries ago. There is an increase in consumer awareness of their own health and health-care costs. Evidence-based science is emerging, linking diet to chronic disease reduction and other health problems or concerns. Certainly, there's a striving for a personalized approach to nutrition, and the new wave of the future, food for the treatment of health conditions.

Do we have any regulation of functional foods? Now, certainly, the primary goal of the FDA is to provide information on labels to consumers about their diet and health. But there is no specific regulatory framework for foods that are being marketed as functional. This movement is just too new. Now, again, keep in mind, however, that if a claim is made, a drug claim is made, for example, a company that is marketing functionality would be prohibited from saying, "cranberry juice prevents bladder infections." They can't say that, but again, as long as they're just marketing or advertising that cranberries are a great source of these wonderful plant-based pigments, again, they're not going to be prohibited from doing that. So it is confusing for the consumer to sort through the information and decide whether it's accurate or not, and whether or not it is worth the additional money.

This is because claims for the health benefit, things such as "now a low-glycemic cereal," or "Contains resveratrol," which is going to be found in red wine and grape juice, or "enriched with DHA, an omega-3 fatty acid" is on the front of the package labeling, it's not a part of the food label. Again, defining the nutrients, so again, if I'm going to the grocery store and I see a margarine that says, "now has stanol esters" all they're doing is defining a nutrient that's in the food that's not required to be part of the food label. Again, defining a nutrient and making a health claim are distinctly different claims on that front of the package.

A survey has found that consumers regard the scientific evidence and other positive aspects of the product containing an unqualified claim similar to those that have an actual qualified, valid structure/function claim. What does this mean? This means that the average consumer can't tell the difference between fact and fiction, and this is why consumers need to understand the concept of a qualified health claim. It's also why the FDA must scrutinize the claims as well. So again, if a company's going to make a claim, a qualified health claim for a food, the FDA will step in and make some kind of ruling on it. The challenge is again, if I just define the nutrient that's being added and stop short of making a claim, there is no governmental regulation.

Currently, there are three claim categories that can be used, and some we've explored in other lectures. There's certainly the nutrient content claim, claim on a food that directly states or implies the level of a nutrient in the food. However, this doesn't make it a health claim, but rather states the nutrient content. So things like low fat, reduced fat, sugar free are all examples. Certainly, there can be a structure/function claim. It gives the role of a nutrient or a dietary ingredient in affecting normal structure or function in humans. However, there's a key distinction that has to be made here. A structure claim does not imply disease prevention, so for example, this structure/function claim could be something like "calcium builds strong bones." That is true, but they cannot say, "calcium prevents osteoporosis." Certainly, a company can say, "fiber enhances bowel regularity." This is true, but they can't make the jump to a disease, "fiber prevents constipation."

Certainly, conventional foods and conventional food manufacturers are not required to notify the FDA about their structure/function claim. For example, milk ads can claim calcium benefits of milk. Health claims on food packaging, and probably there's going to be more controversy seen in this category. Health claims are ways to entice health-seeking consumers to purchase foods, and so companies are routinely petitioning the FDA regarding a new qualified health claim. So again, if a consumer really wants to know if I buy this product, can calcium prevent bone loss? Can it prevent a disease?

And so when the Nutrition Labeling and Education Act was passed in 1990, the FDA initially authorized seven health claims on foods. Manufacturers today can petition the FDA for any health claim that the company believes is valuable, and the key point here is what the current science is going to support. So a sample of such claims would include calcium and osteoporosis, sodium and high blood pressure, fruits and vegetables and cancer, folate and neural tube defects, dietary sugar alcohols and dental caries, and soy protein and heart disease.

However, to make this claim and have this appear on a package, companies have to provide, and the FDA has to review, the strength of the evidence for the claims that are based on all studies that are significant, as well as expert opinions in the field, things such as clinical trials, meta-analysis. So again, it can't be that one study suggested that calcium promotes body fat loss. There really has to be the strength of evidence through a clinical trial or a meta-analysis to very rigorous research design tools to say, yes, the strength of evidence supports this. Certainly, they can provide *in vitro* and *in vivo* studies, as well as numerous literature reviews and searches on well known and reputable studies related to the topic. So when you see these kinds of claims on packages that say, "25 grams of soy protein can aid in the reduction of cardiovascular disease" please know that that manufacturer, as well as the FDA, partnered to review the strength of evidence to say, "I can actually make that claim on food."

Some of the petitions submitted to the FDA for review are accepted, and you might be happy to know that some of the claims are actually denied. So for example, claims related to lutein, and remember, lutein is going to be one of those yellow pigments that are going to be found most visibly in corn. It's in spinach, but it's masked by the chlorophyll. So claims relating lutein to age-related macular degeneration have been denied in recent years, not because there's not some studies saying that they work, but they've been denied based on the strength of the evidence. Again, it's not that the evidence doesn't exist, but rather, it's the type of research study and the determination of a successful endpoint. For instance, what would this be for age-related macular degeneration, the prevention of blindness and the progression of disease? So we are looking at, okay, what's my successful endpoint here? So again, if I'm looking at age-related macular degeneration, do I have to prove that it actually prevents blindness, or would a reduction in the progression of AMD be acceptable? Again, that agreed-upon endpoint is very important. If you want to keep current on the status of these claims, and some claims are approved and some are denied, you can visit the FDA website and type in functional foods, or you can type in qualified health claim.

Cause and effect. Controversial issues arise with functional food in establishing a cause and effect relationship, and why is that the case? It's because many factors can influence food behaviors and mechanism in the human body. It is hard to determine if the food causes the positive effect because it could be related to something else. It could be related to genetics. It could be related to environment. It could be others that have played a role in disease prevention. So for example, would a food prevent diabetes in someone who's lean versus someone who's overweight? There are lots of other confounding variables that make this a little bit difficult to do.

Stricter guidelines should be in place to determine whether these health claims are really helping consumers or if they're adding to the confusion. In addition, will these functional ingredients all behave the same way? Omega-3 fatty acids, for example, are susceptible to oxidation, so are they going to behave the same way in margarine versus juices versus a cereal? Again, I think that science is still evolving. As consumers begin to buy into these functional foods, it's the job of the FDA and nutrition professionals like myself to ensure that the consumer is provided with the correct information. Again, always, always think about a whole food approach.

Frequently asked questions. As a health-care professional and a mother, do you buy foods with functionality in mind? How much weight do I as a dietician give claims to these food? Well, first and foremost, I tend to look at the whole food and not an individual ingredient because we eat foods and not ingredients. But let me tell you what I may do. Say for example, I have a client who absolutely does not like coldwater fish. Coldwater fish, as you might remember, are a great source of omega-3 fatty acids. Or they have a seafood allergy and can't consume coldwater fish. I might help him discover in the food supply some of these functional foods where they've actually added some omega-3 fatty acids to them.

For example, you can manipulate the omega-3 fatty acid content of eggs by what you feed the chicken. So I might have them turn towards a DHA modified egg in order to get some of their really beneficial omega-3 fatty acids. But keep in mind that since the science doesn't tell us if it will behave the same way in an egg as it would in a coldwater fish, I probably would direct them to more than one different source to make sure that we don't have an overreliance on a food where the bioavailability of DHA may not be as strong.

How do I integrate functional foods into my family's diet? Is there a good place to begin? Well, although it seems like sometimes we need to eat mounds of food, the bottom line is you can actually think, okay, I'm going to go back to simple plate organization. What I'm going to do is choose my fruits and vegetables through the colors of the rainbow. That is a really great place to integrate naturally occurring functional foods into the diet. Again, if that's not something that your family's going to buy into, you already eat a lot of fruits and vegetables, is there something else that you can do? Again, sometimes you can look at margarines and other cereals to see whether or not they have some functional ingredients added to them.

I hear all the time, do I really have to eat mounds of healthy foods to acquire all the nutritional benefits? You know what, here's where common sense has to prevail. Keep in mind that your body needs to have a wide variety of nutrients, and we can't cram all these nutrients into a 24-hour environment. So what do we do? Maybe one day, you get something that has yellow in it, and your plate's dominated by yellow. Well, the next day, you just pick another color. Or even more importantly, maybe what you're doing is picking what's seasonal in your area. Keep in mind that over a period of time, maybe not within that 24-hour window, but over a period of time, you're going to get enough of these wonderful good nutrients in your food. Keep in mind, we have to watch our calorie intake. And so I think the challenge is, does the advent of functional foods help our situation, or does it muddy the waters?

I always say, whole foods first, and then if you want to fortify your food supply with some functionality, that's great. So let me go back and answer the question, should you go out and buy those really expensive exotic berry juices? Well, here's a tip for you. If the blues and the reds are what confer the benefit, maybe you want to have grape juice or cranberry juice at a meal, and save your money for that greater whole food approach.

Thank you very much.

A Look at Herbal Therapy
Lecture 30

Optimum nutrition, disease prevention, and wellness, sometimes called "complementary care," are all concepts that resonate with many Americans.

Reasons for the use of herbal therapies are varied and include dissatisfaction with traditional medicine, the need to take charge of your own health care, and the belief that natural medicine is somehow safer than traditional medications. This lecture will explore the myths and realities of herbal medicine with an emphasis on a few of the most popular supplements. Let's explore the intricacies of herbal medicine and try to determine whether it is a healer or a hoax.

A study showed that from 1997 to 2002 there was an increase of herbal therapy use from about 12% to 18.6%. This means around 38 million Americans are using some form of herbal therapy. The predictors of use include being female; having an annual income greater than $65,000 a year; and having greater than a high school education—but users also include the uninsured. The popularity of herbal supplements is often media driven, so the list of the most popular herbal therapies shifts frequently.

Around 38 million Americans are using some form of herbal therapy.

Let's explore the Dietary Supplement Health and Education Act. In the early 1990s, the FDA decided to weigh in on the emerging interest in herbs as medicine. In 1994, the Dietary Supplement Health and Education Act passed, which allowed supplements to be marketed as "all-natural." This act left us with a structure/function claim and a significant number of loopholes.

The unintended consequence of this legislation is that a company does not have to prove that an herbal product is safe before it reaches the market. Products that are contaminated, contain too much of an active ingredient, or contain undeclared substances can reach the market. FDA and consumer reports have found that 49 weight loss pills had undeclared substances. In the United States, removal of products or herbs from the market is rare. Unfortunately, oftentimes it takes a high-profile individual being injured, hurt, or killed.

What about popular supplements and current concerns? The banning of ephedra increased the use of bitter orange for weight loss; in combination with caffeine, it is demonstrated to promote weight loss, but there are drug interactions and side effects. St. John's Wort is used to manage mild to moderate depression but is ineffective for significant depression. Drug interactions and side effects may be significant. *Echinacea* is used to stimulate the immune system. Some experts recommend against it for those with asthma or allergies. Drug interactions may occur with immunosuppressive medications.

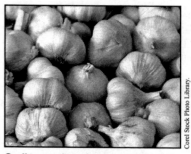

Garlic was thought to lower cholesterol, but it may not be effective.

Garlic was traditionally used to lower cholesterol; however, it may not be effective. There is also a significant risk of bleeding if you use garlic with nonsteroidal anti-inflammatory drugs. Aloe vera is effective topically to promote healthy skin, but aloe latex is a strong laxative and can cause potassium depletion and kidney failure. Oral aloe vera may be effective for treating ulcerative colitis, but there are possible drug interactions.

Gingko biloba's leaves contain flavonoids and compounds that reduce blood clotting, so you should avoid it prior to surgery. Some parts of the plant are beneficial, and some are poisonous. There are possible drug interactions.

Ginseng is a multipurpose herb with various species. Ginseng may thin the blood and act synergistically with other herbs and medicines, so avoid it prior to surgery. As with other herbs, interactions may occur.

Let's review some frequently asked questions. Why is the FDA so opposed to the use of herbal medicines? The FDA is not opposed to their use but would like more information on purity, safety, and efficacy. Are there any labels you should look for to determine if an herbal supplement is safe? Yes, the NSF International seal, the ConsumerLab seal, and the Informed Choice seal. ■

Suggested Reading

Mahan and Stump, *Krause's Food, Nutrition, and Diet Therapy*, chap. 19.

Questions to Consider

1. Has this lecture changed your views about herbal therapies, their use, and their effectiveness? If so, how?

2. Why is it so important to tell your health-care professional not just about herbal therapies you are taking but about supplements you use?

A Look at Herbal Therapy
Lecture 30—Transcript

Greetings, and welcome back. In this lecture, we're going to explore the intricacies of herbal medicine and come to a conclusion, or maybe not, about whether it is a healer or a hoax. In my clinical practice, I had a young adolescent who was really interested in weight loss, and she came to the clinic and told us she was using a popular herbal therapy at the time called MetaboLife. We warned her about some of the potential side effects, but she was going to use this product. She came in one morning not feeling very great, and we'd been monitoring blood pressure and things like that for her. But she came in one morning and didn't feel well. So the nurse practitioner took her blood pressure, and it was 240 over 120. Her heart rate was 170 beats a minute, and we ended up transporting her to a local hospital to have her stomach pumped.

What was the problem? She'd been on this product with really no adversity, and now all of a sudden was having an adverse reaction. Well, the amount of active ingredient in the product that she had switched to, she had opened a new bottle that day, was 200% of what was declared on the label. So it wasn't necessarily the ephedra in that product, but it was the amount of ephedra. So we've got a little bit of a conundrum here on how do we help to navigate this world of herbal therapies? Well, I want to start out by just mentioning that optimum nutrition, disease prevention, and wellness, sometimes called "complementary care," are all concepts that resonate with many Americans. So my young adolescent was really trying to manage her weight issue, and really wanted to manage it on her own and not rely on her physician.

Because these concepts resonate with Americans, herbal therapies and integrative medicine, which is medicine that treats the whole person and his or her lifestyle, that encompasses the physical, psychological, and spiritual self are increasing in popularity. Herbal therapy is oftentimes considered part of the complementary care movement. Interestingly, in the United States, we call herbal therapy oftentimes "alternative medicine," where the rest of the world, where nuts and berries have been used as drugs for centuries, considered it actually traditional medicine.

In my experience, individuals who are interested in complementary medicine are motivated and focused on the prevention and optimum management of disease. They are interested in protecting their health. But when we explore reasons for the use of herbal therapies here in the United States, they're varied, and they include some dissatisfaction with traditional medicine, the need for a patient to take charge of their own health care, and how many of us do that on a regular basis? We want to be more involved. We want to know why a particular medication would be used. Is there a different medication with fewer side effects? There's also a belief that natural medicine is somehow safer than traditional medicines, and so that might drive someone to try an herbal therapy.

In this lecture, we'll explore the myths and realities of herbal medicine in the United States, with an emphasis on some of the few, most popular supplements. Well, let's take a look at the prevalence of use in the United States. This was revealed in a study where David Eisenberg of Harvard and others compared the use of various types of complementary and alternative medicine in 1997 to their use in 2002. What did this study show? It showed an increase in this time period of herbal therapy from about 12% to 18.6%. This represents actually around 38 million Americans who are using some form of herbal therapy. Who are those 38 million Americans?

The predictors of use include being female, an annual income of greater than $65,000 a year, and greater than a high school education. But it also includes the uninsured. Now, why would an uninsured person fall into that same predictor category? Individuals who are under- or uninsured are oftentimes first generation from a foreign country. So in my experience in Houston, many of my immigrant families are using what they consider to be traditional medicines that they bought in Mexico or Central or South America. Oftentimes, they are using what they consider to be traditional, where the other predictors of use really tend to be individuals that might have been born and raised here in the United States.

The popularity of herbal supplements, like what is hot, is oftentimes media-driven. So the list of the most popular herbal therapies shifts frequently. I can remember when everybody was using St. John's Wort, or everybody was using garlic, and again, it's almost the herbal therapy de jour. What is out there and what is popular?

What is different here? What is different about herbal therapy in the United States? I think we need to set the stage by actually exploring the Dietary Supplement Health and Education Act. In the early 1990s, the FDA decided to weigh in on a popular trend, where there was an emerging interest in herbs as medicine. We were all familiar with using garlic as a seasoning agent, or maybe oregano or rosemary, but what happening in the shift in consciousness in the United States in the early 1990s, where now we're starting to look at them as drugs? David Kessler, who was the Commissioner of the FDA, said, wait a minute here. We're going to have to look at this. This is not a food use any more. This is now a drug use. And during that period of time, he proposed a more active role for the FDA in the management of this emerging trend of herbs as medicine.

Industry concern was growing, and public campaigns began because the American population really didn't want the FDA weighing in on what they considered to be something that was in the food supply. Why would the FDA need to regulate that? I think a distinction has to be made at this point in time, though. What Kessler was saying at that point in time was he was not trying to label the garlic that you buy in the grocery store, but when the garlic was used in an amount that you would not normally get as a food, could it potentially have drug effects? Should the American consumer be informed?

You can imagine the flurry of legislation that was being crafted at that point in time. What we had proposed was something called the "Dietary Supplement Health and Education Act." What this was designed to do was be a stopgap, that we really didn't want these herbs regulated as medications, but we didn't want no legislation at all. We wanted something in between. The authors of the original legislation included Tom Harkin, who's a Democrat from Iowa, and Orrin Hatch, a Republican from Utah. The significance of these political authors probably needs to be highlighted. Tom Harkin actually believed that his allergies were cured by using bee pollen, and he has been an advocate for health his whole time serving as a legislator. Orrin Hatch comes from the great state of Utah, and that is where most of the supplement companies are housed, or the manufacturing plants are in Utah. So I think they both had a vested interest on either end of the spectrum on why they wanted some legislation to serve as that middle ground.

What it ended up to be was David Kessler then against the supplement industry. Kessler was looking for something and lo and behold, he got it. What we ended up having during this period of time is there were deaths associated with a contaminated amino acid, L-tryptophan, caused by taking this tainted supplement. It really wasn't the tryptophan, but something that was in the tryptophan supplement. Kessler was saying, wait a minute. This is not an amino acid. This isn't a food any more. We're labeling it differently. We're putting it in a pill or a capsule. Lo and behold, he got some ammunition.

During that period of time, there were supplements on the market, and I remember going into health food stores in Houston and seeing supplements that were claiming to cure HIV, driving individuals away from their primary health-care provider to something in the health food store that was going to cure something which at that point in time was an incurable disease. So you can imagine the flurry of individuals trying to buy supplements to cure their HIV.

Kessler's weighing in on this and saying, we've got a problem. There are some tainted supplements. There are some claims being made. Certainly, during this period of time, opposition came from what was called the Nutritional Health Alliance and Gerald Kessler, no relation to David Kessler. Gerald Kessler hired celebrities to market the herbal industry in commercials. So Whoopi Goldberg was part of this, James Coburn, and Mel Gibson. I remember seeing a commercial, and maybe you saw some of these as well, where Mel Gibson was standing in front of his food pantry with locks on it and saying that what the FDA wanted to do was make all vitamins and minerals and all herbal supplements prescription only. Honestly, this was a fear-driven campaign. That's not what the FDA was looking to do. What they were looking to do was to, again, provide some safeguards for the American public.

There was actually something called "Blackout Friday" in health food stores in 1993, saying, "sign a petition. We need to inform the FDA we don't want our vitamins and minerals prescription only." Ultimately, David Kessler lost his battle against the industry, and in 1994, the Dietary Supplement Health and Education Act actually passed. This allowed supplements to be marketed as all natural, and Americans today embrace this concept. Now, what's the alternative here? Are we going to market them as all fake? Are we going to market them as synthetic? So almost anything that's labeled "all natural" on a product, American consumers are driven to this. So I've always joked that if I was marketing tobacco, I would put waving fields of all-natural tobacco on a cigarette carton and I would call it an all-natural product, and I could do that. You must be aware that there's no legal definition of "all-natural." There is for "organic," but there's not for "all-natural."

What did we end up getting with this concept of the Dietary Supplement Health and Education Act? What we end up with is something called a "structure/function claim." So a dietary supplement can say something about this food, which contains calcium, may promote bone health. So it can make a link between what the compound is and bone health. But it can't say, "calcium cures osteoporosis." It can make a structure/function claim. Another example would be a product could say, "may strengthen the immune system," but it cannot say, "will cure HIV." So this was what the intent was, but unfortunately, the actuality is that we have significant loopholes.

I have on my desk back in Houston ads in trade magazines that violate this over and over and over again. I have one ad that's in a very popular magazine on alternative health care that talks about taking an herbal medication to cure impotence, regardless of its cause, diabetes, heart disease, whatever. It cannot legally do that, but the challenge is there's not adequate numbers of inspectors within the FDA and the FTC, which handle the false advertising, to make sure that these advertisements are actually removed. So I call this "quick kill nutrition." A manufacturer can go in and violate DSHEA, as it's called, the Dietary Supplement Health and Education Act, but by the time they're caught, they've already made a lot of money and pulled out of the market.

Unfortunately, what that means is that we can have dangerous or adulterated or falsely advertised products that reach the market. Concerns also exist for herbal medicines or raw ingredients that might come from China or other foreign countries. Concerns have been raised about the purity of the raw materials, and whether or not some of the raw materials can actually be adulterated with prescription pharmaceuticals. If I'm taking an all-natural herbal product, say for example, valerian, which is marketed to calm me down, if this has been adulterated with valium, I'm going to be really calm. But it's not going to be because of the valerian, but because of the valium. So the United States, being relatively proactive to try and counter this, has opened up a testing facility in China to test the herbal medicines before they reach the United States market. Or more importantly, before the raw ingredients reach the United States market.

What was the unintended consequence of this legislation? We know that it was allowed to make structure/function claims and couldn't make a disease claim, but what was the unintended consequence of this legislation? What we have now is no premarket approval. So in other words, a company does not have to prove that it's safe before it reaches the market. There doesn't have to be a safety study done. Think about this from a pharmaceutical standpoint. Would you want to take a prescription medication where the manufacturer didn't have to tell you the consequences, didn't have to prove that it was safe? You probably wouldn't want that product. Yet in the dietary supplement realm, you can actually buy products with no premarket approval.

The burden of safety has shifted, therefore, from the manufacturer—the manufacturer doesn't have to prove that it's safe—to the FDA, which has to prove that it's unsafe. Now, keep in mind that the FDA doesn't have any more regulators than it did before this legislation passed. This is another concept of saying, yes, we've got legislation on the books. The FDA just needs to enforce it. All true, but if the FDA does not have any more inspectors and they can't do their job because now they're inundated, we've got the legislation. We just lack the enforcement.

Contaminated products or products with too much of the active ingredient, like my poor girl taking MetaboLife, or an undeclared substance, can reach the market. MetaboLife is a great case example. We can argue that low-dose ephedra is unbelievably effective as a weight loss aid. However, if products can have zero ephedra up to 200% of what's declared on the label, we don't have enough safety nets there to control that. Starcaps is a weight loss pill. Six professional NFL football players within the last year, and we've discussed this in an earlier lecture, ended up taking Starcaps as a weight loss aid, and it had an undeclared diuretic on the label. Certainly, FDA and consumer reports have also indicated that of the 61 popular weight loss pills on the market, 49 had an undeclared substance. Keep in mind that if you buy a weight loss product at the health food store that says "All natural" that you may actually be taking a prescription pharmaceutical, and if you're drug-tested, you may not want to have an adverse outcome with that.

In the United States, and here's a key distinction, removal of products or herbs from the market is rare. That is not true in other countries of the world. In other countries, and I'll tell you from my opinion, Germany leads the world in this effort, they have removed products that don't work or are not safe or have adverse outcomes associated with it. So I think the challenge is other countries of the world that look at herbal therapy more as traditional medicine realize and respect that sometimes these medications may need to be removed from the market. And lo and behold, we've currently removed one from the market, and that's ephedra.

Ephedra gained national attention when a pitcher came to training camp, and I will tell you he was overfat and not in great shape. He was taking ephedra for weight loss. What ended up happening is he took more and more of the product. He actually had a heat-related injury and at the time of his death, his core body temperature was reported to be greater than 108 degrees. The way I describe it he cooked from the inside out. So ephedra was then removed from the market. The challenge is, was it the ephedra or was it the dose of the ephedra?

Unfortunately, this is oftentimes what it takes, is when a high profile individual is injured, hurt, killed, maimed from a dietary supplement. That tends to get our attention. Kicker Vencill was a 24-year-old swimmer from Kentucky. He took a multivitamin contaminated with an anabolic steroid that was not declared on the label. So what happened to Kicker? He was banned from swimming. He sued the supplement manufacturer in state court and was awarded over $578,000. But I will tell you what happens to athletes that are caught with a ding on their record. They're looked at as cheaters, and maybe they are, rather than saying, could this young man have possibly known that he was going to test positive for an anabolic steroid when he was taking a multivitamin? I can't look into his mind or into a crystal ball, but I would tell you he probably wouldn't have thought a multivitamin is going to cost him his swimming career.

Another very popular example, and I still have athletes today that want to use this product, is ZMA. This is a dietary supplement with research demonstrating it could significantly increase strength. There was one study demonstrating the effectiveness, and this came from the lab of Victor Conte of the Balco lab scandal. Conte has been considered by some to be the mastermind in the surge in anabolic steroid use by slightly altering the steroid molecule. So we saw high profile Olympians be stripped of their gold medals by being associated with the Balco scandal and some of the anabolic steroid use. So, with ZMA, it was only his research that showed ZMA was going to significantly increase strength. Other research studies following his couldn't prove that it had any beneficial effect at all on strength.

What about popular supplements and current concerns? This is where you might want to sit back in your easy chair and take out a pad and paper and take some notes. You know how things go. When we pull one compound off the market, like we did with ephedra, we're looking for something to replace it with, and lo and behold, enter in bitter orange. Bitter orange chemically is ephedra's cousin, so the banning of ephedra increased the use of this product for weight loss.

I'm going to suggest to you there is science to suggest that ephedra combined with caffeine does improve weight loss outcomes, so you can lose a little bit more weight when you partner these. Well, when ephedra was banned, bitter orange jumped in. Now, bitter orange, along with ephedra, can elevate your blood pressure and elevate your heart rate. So I think the challenge is that when one is replaced with another, you've got to be a little bit careful. So in combination with caffeine, bitter orange is demonstrated to promote weight loss, and certainly, that's going to be the manufacturer's claim.

There are drug interactions with ephedra and other prescription medications, and unfortunately, because these are labeled as supplements, they don't have to declare this on the label. So there's a drug interaction if you happen to be taking an alpha or a beta blocker. There's going to be an interaction with ephedra. MAO inhibitors have an interaction with ephedra, and again, where are you as the consumer going to informed of these interactions unless you're going to a pharmacist or you're seeing a registered dietician on a regular basis?

What are the side effects? Certainly, elevated heart rate and blood pressure, and truly, that's one of the reasons why ephedra and bitter orange help you to lose weight. They actually raise your metabolic rate, and in this case, it's evidenced by an increased heart rate. But what happens if you want to go to sleep at night? If I have an elevated heart rate, an elevated metabolic rate, elevated blood pressure, I may not be able to sleep at night. Certainly, case reports exist of a stroke in an otherwise healthy 38-year-old male taking ephedra and taking some of these weight loss products. So again, you have to be a little bit careful. Was it the herb in there? Was it an adulterated pharmaceutical? Was this individual taking a pharmaceutical along with a prescription medication? You've got to be a little bit of a nutrition detective before you're going to venture into this world.

St. John's Wort. The major use of this herb is for the management of mild to moderate depression. The problem is the results from major studies are inconclusive. Some say it works, and some say it doesn't. Many of these studies indicate this herb might be effective for minor or mild depression. However, a major clinical trial for major depression concluded that St. John's Wort is ineffective for significant depression. Now, I'm going to mention this more than once because I think it's a key point. In the countries of the world that get this right, if you have an illness or a condition that really does require a pharmaceutical, you would be discouraged from taking a less effective herbal medication.

The drug interactions with St. John's Wort may be significant, and this is one of these herbs that you saw splashed all over the newspaper, and then all of a sudden, it started to contract and lost a little bit of favor. It's because it interferes with many drugs. It can interfere with birth control pills. That might be an unintended consequence that you weren't looking for. But if you've had something like a kidney transplant, any kind of organ transplant, and you are on lifelong immunosuppressive therapy, it will reduce the effectiveness of those drugs. It can interfere with warfarin, which is an anticoagulant.

It can interfere with digoxin, which is used to treat some heart problems. It can also cause mania in those with an underlying mood disorder. Now, keep in mind when St. John's Wort first came out, we had no warning of those side effects because there was no need for premarket approval. So all of this was discovered in individuals just like you, just like me, who went out and took these, and all of a sudden, had an adverse reaction.

What about Echinacea? Echinacea is one of those herbs that is used to stimulate the immune system. Some studies suggest that Echinacea is effective for the treatment of upper respiratory infections. And again, we're always going to find there are some studies, not all studies. Some experts recommend against the use of Echinacea for autoimmune disorders, such as lupus, and TB. Why might that be the case? If Echinacea actually stimulates the immune system, and you have an autoimmune disorder like lupus, with an immune system that's out of kilter, you may not want something that's going to stimulate your immune system.

As with most herbal therapies, it's a plant, so it's part of the Aster family. Keep in mind that if you're highly allergic to a particular plant, if the herb you're going to take is in the same botanical family, this might be a contraindication. Those with significant asthma or allergies outside of this plant family should really probably avoid this preparation as well. Additionally, for those with an immunoglobulin E mediated hypersensitivity, there is an increased risk of anaphylaxis, the ability to move air and where you stop breathing. A study, however, evaluating the amount and the correct species in health food stores revealed very disappointing results. Ten percent of the products tested had absolutely no Echinacea. Forty-three percent of the products tested met the standards listed on the label.

The claims of a standardization of an extract listed on an herbal therapy, and oftentimes you'd find that on the front of the label, are not insurance. Now, I want you to think about this. If very few or 10% of those herbal medications had no active ingredient, you've wasted your money, or you switch brands and you increase the dose, and now you have an adverse reaction because you took too much of it. Also, within this family, possible interactions may also occur with immunosuppressive medications.

Garlic was traditionally used to lower cholesterol, and it is a common prescription in Germany. So if your cholesterol is mildly elevated and you go to a German physician, he or she may try garlic first, and then ramp it up if your cholesterol's not well controlled. A recent meta-analysis suggested that although garlic was more effective than placebo, the amount of cholesterol reduction was modest. Here's another example. If your total cholesterol is 400, garlic is not going to be effective enough for you to have significant cholesterol reduction. Garlic was also used as an antimicrobial agent during both World Wars, and it's relatively effective. However, there's a significant risk of bleeding that exists if you use garlic with non-steroidal anti-inflammatory drugs, such as aspirin, Aleve, Motrin, and other drugs that affect blood clotting, including other herbs, such as gingko biloba.

What about aloe vera? Do you all have an aloe vera plant in your yard? I certainly do. It has been used topically for centuries to promote healthy skin and it's effective for this use. Aloe juice can be taken orally. The latex portion of the aloe plant is a very strong laxative and can cause potassium depletion and kidney failure. So keep in mind that aloe latex is not the same thing as aloe vera.

Aloe latex is often sold in foreign countries, and I've seen it available from street vendors in Mexico. In the United States, the FDA required reformulation in 2002 to remove the offending compounds. A small study suggested that oral aloe vera may be effective for treating ulcerative colitis. That has a therapeutic effect as it's swallowed. But further research is needed to confirm this effect. Possible interactions may occur with some medications for diabetes, digoxin and diuretics.

An additional popular herb, gingko biloba, has been used as part of traditional Chinese medicine for centuries, and the leaves contain flavonoids and compounds that reduce blood clotting. Due to its anticoagulant effect, it should be avoided prior to surgery. Now, think of the additive effect here. Gingko, garlic, and omega-3 fatty acids, which we've discussed in the past, all prevent blood clotting. They all have an effect, so you as a consumer need to be aware that if you're taking a combination of different kinds of vitamin supplements and herbs, you might have to discontinue those prior to surgery.

Again, the part of the plant makes it either a benefit or a poison. Gingko biloba seeds can be fatal, and have been associated with seizures in children. So where the plant leaves might be appropriate, the seeds are not. The effectiveness of gingko biloba for intermittent claudication or leg pain or peripheral occlusive artery disease has demonstrated that it actually is effective for reducing pain, probably because it has an anti-inflammatory effect similar to aspirin. But there are possible interactions that might occur with this plant, including interactions with antihypertensive medications, blood sugar lowering medications, anticonvulsant, and antidepressant medications.

What about ginseng? Actually, there is more than one species that is being used for dietary supplements. It's been used medicinally for over 2000 years. Ginseng may actually thin the blood and act synergistically with other herbs and medicines. So this is another one that you want to avoid prior to surgery. It's often reported to be a tonic or adaptogenic herb, indicating it's a multipurpose herb. Siberian ginseng, that specific species, is linked with hypertension, but not the other ginseng species. Reported benefits for exercise performance, improvement in diabetes, again, are all going to be species-specific. Controlling mood, cognitive, and sexual function, studies on those functions have come back with mixed results.

Some of the variability of these studies actually is because of the difference in the species. So again, not all ginseng species are going to act the same way. Certainly, as with other herbs, possible interactions may occur, and again, oftentimes you have those synergistic effects with other herbs that interfere with blood clotting, so blood thinning medications, medications used to treat heart disease, diabetes medication. So what's that prudent use? Tell your primary health-care provider about the use of herbal therapies. Ask your pharmacist about interaction. Don't use for those conditions that require significant pharmacological action, so for cancer and heart disease, diabetes and hypertension. That's not the way these drugs are used in other countries. So if you have a need for significant pharmacotherapy, don't consider herbal therapies as your mainstay.

Frequently asked questions. I come from a country where herbs have been used as nutritional supplements for centuries. Why is the FDA so opposed to their use? In the United States, we do not traditionally remove herbal medicines when there's an adverse reaction. Other countries of the world, such as Germany, do. They remove products. The FDA is not opposed to their use, but would like more information on purity, safety, and efficacy to protect the American consumer.

Are there any labels you should look for to determine if an herbal supplement is safe? Certainly, there's an NSF International seal, a ConsumerLab seal, and Informed Choice. These seals are the consumer's best assurance that a product is not contaminated. I always suggest that those who are interested in purity, safety, and efficacy join Consumer Labs and get safety alerts delivered right to their desktop.

Thank you very much.

Organic or Conventional—Your Choice
Lecture 31

Consumer purchases of organic products have increased by 20% each year, and organic foods have appeared in grocery stores worldwide. Are there significant health benefits to choosing organic foods?

L et's explore the world of organic products. We have to keep things in perspective. A client of mine stopped buying produce because organic produce it was too expensive and she refused to eat anything not organic. So she wound up eating more processed foods. Some 81% of consumers buy organic foods because they believe they have a higher nutritive value than conventional foods.

Organic is a legally defined term that describes the way farmers cultivate and process agricultural products. The term "organic" can be applied to produce, meat, dairy, poultry, and processed foods. Organic produce is designed to support soil and water conservation and reduce pollution. It does not allow for irradiation or genetically modified foods. Organic farmers use natural fertilizers and beneficial insects to reduce pests and diseases. Organically farmed animals are provided with organic feed and no antibiotics or growth hormones. Organically farmed

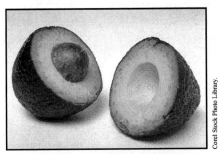

Corel Stock Photo Library.

Avocados are among the foods that contain the lowest levels of pesticides.

animals are allowed to be free range and must be humanely slaughtered. The USDA has guidelines for its organic certification program, but there are no national standards for organic seafood at this time.

Is organic produce more nutritious? Organic foods have fewer nitrates present. High nitrate content may cause methemoglobulinemia; cancers of the digestive tract, bladder, and ovaries; and non-Hodgkin's lymphoma. Omega-6 is considered to be an inflammatory fatty acid and has been linked to eczema. Conventional milk has higher omega-6 than organic. Studies have shown that organic crops contain more vitamin C, polyphenolic compounds, essential amino acids, total sugars, alpha-tocopherol, and phosphorus than conventional crops. Conventional food samples had equivalent amounts of beta-carotene, yet higher levels of potassium, compared to organic food samples. Crude protein was significantly higher in the conventionally grown wheat product.

The foods that contain the most residual pesticides are peaches, apples, sweet bell peppers, celery, nectarines, strawberries, cherries, pears, grapes, spinach, lettuce, and potatoes.

There are always concerns about pesticides. Pesticide consumption has been linked to solid tumor cancers, non-Hodgkin's lymphoma, and leukemia, as well as some childhood cancers. Organic foods have lower levels of pesticides than conventional foods. Dietary intake is the most common source of pesticide levels in the human body. The overall amount of pesticides on any fruit or vegetable poses a very small health risk to adults, but it can be a concern in children.

The foods that contain the most residual pesticides are peaches, apples, sweet bell peppers, celery, nectarines, strawberries, cherries, pears, grapes, spinach, lettuce, and potatoes. Foods that contain the least amount of pesticides are papaya, broccoli, cabbage, bananas, kiwi, mangoes, pineapple, avocados, and onions.

So where does this leave us? The USDA does not claim that organic products are more nutritional than conventional products. No conclusive evidence suggests that organic foods are beneficial in the prevention of diseases or common health concerns. Organic foods may spoil faster because they have no preservatives. The bottom line is that you should follow personal preferences and your own opinion. Organic produce can cost 10%–30% more than conventional foods. Organic animal products and processed foods may be up to 100% more expensive. This is because they are much more labor intensive.

Tips for consumers: Buy fresh produce in season; read labels; thoroughly wash both organic and conventional produce; if you are concerned about conventional fruits and vegetables, peel them.

Let's review some frequently asked questions. Are there certain times in the life cycle when eating organic is particularly important? In general, the more vulnerable the population, the greater the advantage to choosing organic.

Do vegetable washes and sprays remove all pesticides? Scrubbing fruits and vegetables with water for at least 30 seconds may be just as effective as washes.

If we prefer but cannot afford organic, should we just skip the fresh fruits and vegetables and take a multivitamin instead? No, fruits and vegetables have phytochemicals that pills do not. ∎

Suggested Reading

Burke, *To Buy or Not to Buy Organic.*

Questions to Consider

1. What are the factors you consider when determining whether to purchase organic products?

2. Why do you think the demand for organic products has increased in recent years?

Organic or Conventional—Your Choice
Lecture 31—Transcript

Hello, and welcome back. I'm going to tell you a story about a family that I had that was really trying to make a good decision, but it was better defined as a good decision gone bad. I was working with a family who we were really trying to promote a plant-based diet, and the mom came in and said, "you know what, I stopped buying produce." I said, "Well, why did you stop buying produce?" And she said, "because I can't afford apples that are $3.50 a pound that are organic, and so if it's not organic, I won't eat it." She gave up buying fruits and vegetables. So what did she substitute it for? Well, she was buying more snack foods and more processed foods, and again, the intent was, "I want to provide healthy food for my family," but kind of missed the boat.

We're going to explore a little bit about the world of organic products and a little bit on choosing between organic and conventional. Well, let's take a little bit of a look at organic products and what consumers are doing. Consumer purchases of organic products have increased by 20% each year. That's pretty significant. These organic foods have been introduced into many grocery stores worldwide, so you used to only be able to find them in specialty stores or health food stores, and now almost every grocery store chain is going to have its own line of organic.

The Food Marketing Institute estimates that about 50% of all shoppers in the United States have bought at least one organic product. So again, keep in mind that as this becomes mainstream, sales actually go up because you can get all your food in one store. Even more so, 81% of consumers surveyed buy organic foods because they believe it has a higher nutritive value than conventional foods. Now, we'll explore if it really does, or if this is marketing. Many consumers believe that these foods can help to prevent certain diseases and reduce health risks, so they are willing to pay the extra price for organic.

But, are there significant health benefits to choosing organic foods? Are there nutritional concerns and qualified research supporting organic versus conventional? And this will ultimately come down to your personal choice.

Which way do you want to take your family? Well, these questions must be answered, as global organic sales increase. Although the numbers indicate that sales are going to continue to increase, do consumers have any idea what they're actually putting into their shopping carts? Or are they going to make the same kind of error that my client did, if it's not organic, it's not for me?

This lecture will explain the terms of what defines an organic product, and what the current research has discovered regarding organic foods in the marketplace. So again, let's start out with our basic definitions. What is an organic food? "Organic" is actually a legally defined term, and it describes the way farmers cultivate and process agricultural products. It is also designed to support soil and water conservation and reduce pollution, so for you as a consumer, that may be enough of a reason to choose organic produce.

It also will not allow for irradiation or genetically modified foods. That cannot be certified as "organic." Additionally, farmers do not use conventional methods to fertilize or prevent crop diseases. They use natural fertilizers, such as manure or compost. Keep in mind that manure can contain *E. coli* and if they're using a true manure product, you have to wash organic products just like you do conventional. Additionally, organic products use beneficial insects to reduce pests and diseases. Animals are provided with organic feed and no antibiotics or growth hormones can be used in the raising or cultivating of that crop.

Allowance of free range. Animals are not cooped up in a pen, but I want to caution you here for a second. We have to sort out, is this marketing or is this science? When you look at what happens with chickens, chickens at birth need to be imprinted, and what that means is that they follow along with what the rest of the crowd does, and that becomes their behavior. So if a young chicken is not allowed to be out of the coop, or is not out of the coop very early in life, they're actually afraid of going out into the yard. And so they're allowed free range. That's the key word there. They're allowed free range, but it doesn't necessarily mean they will be free range. Additionally, animals that are processed in an organic way must be humanely slaughtered.

The term "organic" cannot be applied only to produce and meat and dairy foods and poultry, but also to processed foods that include breakfast cereals, crackers, baby foods, and the like. The USDA has guidelines for its organic certification program. Before a label can be given, a government-approved certifier must inspect the farm to make sure that the farmer follows all the rules. So again, this is our first guarantee. The symbol or label is a green and white circle, with the words "USDA organic" and so that's what you're looking for. Again, this is oftentimes front-of-package labeling.

The USDA gives regulations on how foods are grown, handled, and processed, so it makes sense that they're involved with this process. Any organic food manufacturer or farmer that claims to sell organic products must have it labeled as USDA certified, unless—there's always that exception to the rule—they sell less than $5000 per year in organic foods. So again, you may have a wonderful organic farmer in your neighborhood that you buy from on a regular basis, but none of his or her products would have to have that label if they sell less than $5000 a year in organic foods.

What about the labels? What kinds of words can we look for on those labels? Well, "100% organic," what does that mean? It means it's a completely organic product and made from all organic ingredients, and this can bear the green and white USDA label. "Organic" is another thing that you can see on the label, and at least 95% of the product is organic. Again, it can bear the same green and white label. How does something become 95% organic? This is usually a product with more than one ingredient, like bread or pasta. You also might see it on a mixed fruit dish or something like yogurt, so again, almost everything is organic, but not quite.

Then we have "Made with organic ingredients." The product contains at least 70% organic ingredients, and a lot of the energy bars that are on the market are going to have this seal. So you can go and say, "well, I'm going to buy a sports bar to go run," and you see the 70% organic ingredients. The organic seal cannot be used on this package, so you won't see the white and green circle. "All natural," "free range," and "hormone free"—these labels should not be confused with "organic." Those aren't necessarily legally protected terms, so be careful with that. Only the foods that meet the USDA standards can receive the organic label.

There are no national standards for organic seafood at this time, and part of it's because we import seafood from other parts of the world. Well, what about the nutritional value? Remember, that's what drives consumers' interest. Consumers believe the nutritional value of organic produce, particularly, is going to be greater than its conventionally grown counterparts. Well, the debate continues to rage whether organic produce is more nutritious, and the focus of the research has been on the following ingredients. So we don't have all the science sorted out, but we've focused in on these following ingredients.

The nitrate content. Nitrate is actually a salt of nitric acid, and it's a naturally occurring compound in some foods. The main contributors of nitrate in the diet include green leafy vegetables and oftentimes drinking water. Nitrogenous fertilizers may also contribute to the higher nitrate content of some foods. And again, this is going to be something that's going to be regulated by the US Environmental Protection Agency. So again, sometimes the nitrate can occur naturally in foods, or it can be a byproduct, something that is not designed to be there. The US Environmental Protection Agency says an acceptable daily intake is less than 10 parts per million. High nitrate content can have negative effects. Now, that does not mean if you're eating a green leafy vegetable with a higher nitrate content that you need to stop. It really is implying those things that become run-off in water.

What does a high nitrate content cause? It causes methemoglobulinemia, which can occur when nitrates, that are not supposed to be in your food supply, directly interact with hemoglobin, making it unable to carry oxygen in infants. So here's an example. When I remove nitrogen fertilizers—and remember, organic food can't have crops grown in conventional ways—I'm removing some of the source of what's considered to be undesirable nitrate in my diet. Well, certainly, this nitrate can also be linked with cancers of the digestive tract, bladder, and ovaries. So again, the nitrate fertilizers, or the nitrogenous fertilizers, may be that initiating event in cancer.

It's also linked with non-Hodgkin's lymphoma. Several studies have been conducted on the levels of nitrates in organic versus conventional foods. There have been mixed results, and again, science usually yields mixed results, with some showing that organic foods have significantly fewer nitrates. Does that make sense? That should make sense because they're not using these forms of fertilizer. However, other studies have shown that conventional food has fewer nitrates. But overall, if we're going to cut to the chase, most studies give evidence that organic foods do have lower numbers or quantities of nitrates present on the foods.

Another nutritional debate in organic versus conventional is the fatty acids in milk, and most of us think that the fat in milk is an animal fat that is really not desirable. So the fatty acids that have been studied include polyunsaturated fats, and particularly omega-3 fatty acids, which, as we know from previous lectures, have positive benefits. Then they compare that and take a look at the omega-6 fatty acid content of milk, which is linked to more negative health outcomes, and oftentimes considered to be an inflammatory fatty acid. The fatty acid profile in milk has been linked to eczema, as organic milk has a higher level of omega-3 fatty acids than omega-6. Conventional milk has higher omega-6. Well, isn't milk just milk? We'll explore that in a little bit more detail.

Organic dairy products have been studied and are associated with a lower risk of eczema in the first two years of life as a child. A research study used milk samples from 19 conventional milk source and 17 organic dairy farms, and here were the results. Organic milk from cows that are mostly grass-fed had a higher percentage of total omega-3 fatty acids versus conventional milk. The conventional milk from corn-fed cows had significantly lower percentages of omega-3, and therefore had little impact on skin disease. Remember, omega-6 fatty acids are inflammatory, may contribute to dermatitis or skin disease, so again, the final verdict here is the fatty acid content of milk, or meat of any animal, is dependent on how the animal was fed. In the United States, most conventionally processed meat and milk are going to be corn-fed, not grass-fed. American consumers are oftentimes a little bit fussy. They don't really like the way grass-fed milk tastes, or grass-fed meat tastes, and again, this is an acquired taste.

What about other things, other than the fatty acid content? What about vitamin C and other nutrients? Well, examples of foods that have been studied to compare conventional versus organic include lettuce, spinach, kale, chard, cabbage, and radishes. The results of one study show that organic crops contain more of the following than conventional crops. More vitamin

C, more of those wonderful polyphenolic compounds that are linked with potential health benefits. For example, the polyphenols in dark chocolate make it a healthy treat in moderation. So again, organic compounds, organic foods, may have more of these wonderful polyphenolic compounds. Essential amino acids and total sugars are also going to be different in organic versus conventional.

Another study analyzed matched pairs of organic and conventional samples, and determined that the vitamin C, the alpha-tocopherol, or a form of vitamin E, and phosphorus were higher in organic samples, as much as 63%, 62%, and 63% respectively. The conventional food samples had equivalent amounts of beta-carotene, that wonderful vitamin A precursor, yet higher levels of potassium compared to organic food samples. The conclusions to be drawn from these studies as to one theory as to why organic foods may have more nutrients is that the shelf life is shorter for organic foods, and therefore they might be fresher.

Keep in mind that organic foods are also not going to have that waxy coating on the outside, so they don't last as long. Organic produce also may be more likely to be more locally grown, and I can tell you, at the stores in Houston, they'll also talk about Texas-grown organic foods to let us know that that organic food didn't have to travel all throughout the United States. And again, the longer it sits on the shelf, you might have some deterioration of nutritional value.

Crude protein can also be different in organic versus conventional. Wheat protein quality and composition of organic versus conventional foods have been compared, and what are the results of wheat protein quality? Crude protein was significantly higher in the conventionally grown wheat product. Why might that be? Scratch our heads and say, what's the cause of that? Well, the thought is that when plants are treated with a nitrogen-rich fertilizer, their protein production is enhanced. If you remember back to the protein lecture, what makes protein unique as opposed to carbohydrate and fat is its nitrogen content. If I'm processing a plant with a nitrogen-rich fertilizer, it should make intuitive sense. Okay, nitrogen equals protein, and the protein content might be higher in conventionally grown wheat.

Organic products also appear not to take up nitrogen as fast as the conventional ones do. Now, although organic products are lower in crude protein, their amino acid profile—and remember, an amino acid is a building block of proteins—may actually be higher than conventional ones, making them a higher quality protein, but less total protein.

Now, what about flavonoids, which are a wonderful group of antioxidants and a wonderful subgroup of this polyphenolic compounds? These are a group of compounds often associated, again, with the pigments in plants. Dried tomato products have been looked at, conventional versus organic, and they've been studied over a 10-year period. So what do we know? What are the results? There were significantly higher levels of three particular flavonoids, quercetin, kaempferol, and naringenin, which were found in the organic tomato samples. So again, higher amounts of polyphenolic compounds.

What about pesticide concerns? There are always concerns about pesticides. Pesticide consumption has controversial effects, and has been shown to be linked to, but not causative, solid tumor cancers, non-Hodgkin's lymphoma and leukemia, as well as some childhood cancers. What about breast cancer and pesticide use? Research has concluded there's really no connection between breast cancer incidences in women living in areas with high levels of agricultural pesticides. So again, when we're thinking about should I or should I not, the question remains, is this a major cause of cancer? I think the jury's still out on this. Organic foods have lower levels of pesticides, when compared to conventional foods.

Keep in mind, however, that trace amounts of pesticides may be in the soil, even though no pesticides were used. So again, organic products may have trace amounts of pesticides, not because the farmer is breaking the law or breaking the standard, but because the soil is going to retain some of those pesticides. Certainly, dietary intake, food, is the most common source of pesticide levels in the human body. The overall amount of pesticides on any fruit or vegetable, whether it's conventional or organic, actually poses a very small health risk to adults. But keep in mind that the result is not zero. The risk is not zero. And therefore the reason many consumers would like to reduce the risk, and get it as close to zero as possible, and possibly increase the nutrition, think, "I'm going to buy organic."

Children can be a concern with high levels of pesticides, particularly organophosphate pesticides, and so organic products may be beneficial in this at-risk population. So you're at the grocery store. You're thinking, okay, I understand it's controversial. Pesticides may not pose a huge risk. Organic food may be a little bit more nutritious, but not for every nutrient. So are there foods that are going to contain more pesticides than others? How am I going to refine my grocery list? Well, the foods that contain the most residual pesticides on the fruit are going to be things like peaches, apples, sweet bell peppers, celery, nectarines, strawberries, cherries, pears, grapes, spinach, lettuce, and potatoes. So those are the big 12. Now, keep in mind that what make those things so unique is that oftentimes you eat the whole plant.

Foods, on the other hand foods that contain the least amount of pesticides, in part because most have skin and outer layers that you don't eat, are things like papaya, but then broccoli. We eat almost all of the broccoli, so that's not universally true. Cabbage, you can always peel off those outer layers on the cabbage plant, bananas, certainly, most people don't eat the peel, kiwi, mangoes, pineapple, avocados, and onions. So if I'm trying to look at my grocery dollar and think, how can I maximize my dollar and do the best job of protecting my health? I'm probably going to stay away from the big 12, but I might buy conventional onions because I'm not concerned as much about the risk.

Organic farming. I think one of the issues is that you can still have a pest and pathogen problem. You can combat this, and farmers can combat this by using crop rotations, and organizing appropriate crop planting times. To minimize pathogens in crops with the use of raw animal manure for fertilization, human consumption must wait at least 120 days between the manure application and the harvest of the crop. Now, I'll tell you, this is a little bit difficult to enforce because a farmer could use raw manure and there's not going to be a certifier that's going to come out and inspect to make sure that they waited 120 days. I think we've had some incidents where organic lettuce has actually been tainted with *E. coli*, probably because they didn't wait that 120 days.

Well, what about the research on the presence of other pathogens? Reports indicate that there was no statistically significant difference in *E. coli* prevalence in certified organic versus conventional produce.

So where does this leave us? Nutrition information. The USDA does not claim that organic products are more nutritious than conventional. Some of the science says yes, and some of the science says no. There's a lot of contradicting evidence and research, as seen from the studies we've explored, on organic versus conventional food products. More extensive long-term research is needed in order to determine that significant nutritional claims can be made about organic products.

What about health concerns? Really, there is no conclusive evidence to suggest that organic foods are beneficial in the prevention of diseases or common health concerns. So we can't say, "If you eat organic produce, you're less likely to have diabetes." There's really no conclusive evidence. There's no long-term data analysis that have proven these results to be conclusive across the board.

What about quality? We do know organic foods may spoil faster, such as fruits and vegetables, because they have no preservatives. I have children, for example, who will look at an organic apple and it looks a little mottled, and they don't like the way it looks. It's not shiny and as red as the normal apples that they get, and so they reject it.

The bottom line is all this is based on personal preference and your own opinion. Which direction do you want to go? Certainly, when we talk about pesticides, the overall levels of pesticides are lower on organic foods than conventional. Now, what about the cost? And this is oftentimes, again, my family that made the wrong decision. Organic produce can cost 10% to 30% more than conventional foods. Animal products and processed foods may be up to 100% more expensive. So again, I think in families that are trying to pinch pennies, you might want to say, "I'm going to avoid the ones that are most likely to be contaminated with pesticides and I'm going to buy conventional with the other produce that is least likely to be contaminated."

Why are these products so much more expensive? Well, they're much more labor intensive. You have to have expensive tools to control weeds, rather than buying pesticides. It's very easy to spread a pesticide. It's not so easy to put in beneficial insects or other kinds of barriers to pathogens and overgrowth of weeds.

Taste. Is taste a difference? Well, there seems to be really no difference in taste among consumers when comparing the two products. So again, it all depends on the taste preference of consumers. I look at this and think it's more a visual issue with consumers than it is a taste issue.

Do we have any tips for consumers? Buy fresh produce in season to receive the highest quality and the best price. Visit local farmers' markets to support local farmers and receive the freshest produce possible. I'm very fortunate that on Tuesdays and Thursdays, the local farmers in south Texas actually have a farmers' market at Rice. All I have to do is walk into the parking lot and I can get organic peaches. Remember, peaches are high in pesticides. I can buy organic peaches that are absolutely mouthwatering. If you have a farmers' market in your area, visit the local farmers' market, make a relationship with the local farmer and ask if they're providing you with organic produce.

Start your own garden or participate in a community garden project as well. Read labels. Has that not been a consistent theme? Read labels carefully and know what you're buying. "Organic" doesn't necessarily mean healthier, especially when we're talking about processed foods. I could buy an organic macaroni and cheese, for example, but that product still could be high in total fat or salt, and depending on the product, it could be high in sugar and calories. So you must read the label. Keep in mind that "organic" doesn't mean that it's lower in calories. You have to read the label. One of the things that you can do with both organic and conventional produce is thoroughly wash it. Scrub the outside if you're going to eat that outside peel.

If you're concerned about conventional fruits and vegetables, peel them. So if you're concerned that your family is eating a conventionally grown apple, high pesticide concern, peel the apple. If pesticides are an issue for you, buy organic produce that is listed on the highest pesticide content list.

Our frequently asked questions. Other than infancy and early childhood, which I've mentioned, are there certain times in the life cycle when eating organic is particularly important? What about pregnancy, chronic illness, and old age? In general, the more vulnerable the population, the greater the advantage to choosing organic. So I would say the bottom line is if you're concerned about pregnancy, and again, we don't have any long-term studies on pesticides and pregnancy outcome, but if you're concerned and you want to do everything possible, go ahead and choose organic. Keep in mind that even though the research isn't there, it might give you the psychological relief to know that you've done everything possible. Same thing with your children—you might want to do that. Again, there is some link between pesticides and certain forms of cancer. Children can be vulnerable, mostly because of their body weight. So children are going to have a higher amount of pesticide per pound of body weight than an adult because they weigh less. So maybe with your children, you think, "I would really like to make sure I'm using organic produce with my children."

What about the vegetable washes and sprays that are available? Don't they remove all pesticides? Well, you know what, that's the claim, but a small study suggests that it's the mechanical action of scrubbing fruits and vegetables with water for at least 30 seconds that's just as effective as the washes. I'll tell you, early on in my clinical practice, I had the very fortunate experience of working with an HIV population. In this population, in addition to scrubbing, we actually suggested that to kill the bacteria—because that was a bigger issue for an HIV population—on fruits and vegetables, that you could take about a teaspoon of bleach. Now, I know that doesn't sound delicious. But a teaspoon of bleach to about a gallon of water, and that will kill the bacteria that are on the food. So that may be a tip for you as well.

Another question that I get is, I like to buy organic, but I just can't afford it. So shouldn't we just skip the fresh fruits and vegetables and make sure we all take a multivitamin? The answer on this is please, no, don't do that. Because again, remember what fruits and vegetables have that a pill will not is the wonderful phytochemicals that are in them, the polyphenolic compounds, the quercetin, the anthocyanins, all these wonderful pigments that are in fruits and vegetables that are not going to be found in a pill. Again, if you're concerned and budget is an issue, peel the ones that are the most suspect, the ones that are on the big 12 list. Peel those, and then, again, choose organic for the other ones. Again, choose the ones that are most likely to be contaminated, peel them, and it's a great way to remove the residue and the wax, but please, don't ever stop eating fruits and vegetables.

The take-home message on this lecture, and this one, again, is a little bit different than the other ones, we don't have all the science that we need to make a definitive conclusion. So it comes down to your budget, your personal beliefs, how many vulnerable populations you have in your family, and again, your own psychological relief by choosing organic versus conventional.

Thank you very much.

Solutions:

Fake or Real—Sugars and Fats
Lecture 32

Numerous products on the market are made with artificial sweeteners, fat replacements, and other additives, which makes it difficult to determine if what we are eating is real or fake.

Your preference for sweetness varies by genetics, exposure during early childhood, and whether you are full or hungry. Nearly a third of the extra sugars we consume are from sugar-sweetened soft drinks.

By definition, a nutritive sweetener is something that is sweet tasting and has energy. The common ones that you are familiar with are sucrose and fructose. These are usually easily digestible. Sugar alcohols are also nutritive sweeteners and include manitol, sorbitol, xylitol, maltitol, and hydrogenated starch. These are generally regarded as safe food additives, but they can cause gas, cramping, bloating, and diarrhea. Foods with sugar alcohols can be labeled "sugar free." They have a reduced glycemic response and dental caries risk and may have a prebiotic effect.

Nonnutritive sweeteners provide a sweet taste but no energy. Five nonnutritive sweeteners currently have FDA approval: acesulfame-K, aspartame, neotame, saccharin, and sucralose. They are anywhere between 160 to many hundreds of times sweeter than sugar and are noncariogenic. Aspartame (a.k.a. NutraSweet) generates a limited glycemic response, but acesulfame-K, neotame, saccharin, and sucralose generate no glycemic reaction. These nonnutritive sweeteners may be beneficial in managing diabetes, controlling weight, and preventing cavities.

Heating does not reduce the sweetening power of acesulfame-K, neotame, saccharin, or sucralose, though prolonged heat may cause a loss of sweetness with aspartame. Saccharin was once labeled as a carcinogen, but in 2000 this was removed from its label.

Both nutritive and nonnutritive sweeteners have very little evidence of detrimental long-term effects on overall health. Caution should be taken during childhood and pregnancy to avoid excessive amounts of nonnutritive sweeteners. The Institute of Medicine says that no more than 25% of calories consumed should be added sugars. Too much sugar in the diet may cause a person to decrease consumption of essential vitamins and minerals needed by the body to function. Excess sugar can contribute to obesity. Nonnutritive sweeteners have the potential to reduce calorie intake.

No more than 25% of calories consumed should be added sugars.

Diabetics may use nonnutritive sweeteners because they do not raise blood sugar. Nutritive sweeteners should not be completely restricted, but they have to be monitored. However, for those with type 2 diabetes, nonnutritive sweeteners can aid in weight control. No relationship has been established between the risk for common cancers or cancerous tumors and sweeteners.

Many processed foods contain fat replacers. These fat replacers must be able to copy some or all of the functional properties of fat. Most of the fat replacers are classified into 3 groups: carbohydrate based, protein based, or lipid based. Carbohydrate-based fat replacers absorb water to form gels that simulate a texture similar to fat. Protein-based fat replacers are made from milk, oftentimes whey protein. Lipid-based fat replacers are fat modified by chemical changes that will inhibit absorption.

Fat extenders generally reduce calories by diluting the fat with water in the form of an oil and water emulsion. Lipid analogs have many characteristics of fat but have a different digestibility and nutritional value.

If the substance is labeled as GRAS (generally regarded as safe), that means the FDA has evidence that it is safe to use in food. However, concerns have been associated with Olestra and polydextrose, both of which have the ability to cause stomach upset. If fat replacers are used in an overall diet plan that promotes the use of healthy fats and a variety of low-fat products, then a balanced calorie intake can be achieved.

Let's review a frequently asked question. How do I use applesauce or fruit purees as replacers in baked goods? Use them to replace about 50% of the oil in the recipe. You can reduce the fat in your foods, but fat-free foods are difficult to achieve. ■

Suggested Reading

Brown, A., *Understanding Food*, chaps. 20–21.

Duyff, *American Dietetic Association Complete Food and Nutrition Guide*, chaps. 3, 5.

Questions to Consider

1. What artificial sweeteners and fat replacers do you regularly use? How would your diet change if you could not buy artificial sweeteners or fat replacers?

2. Despite our increased use of these lower-calorie products, the American waistline is still expanding. Why?

Lecture 32: Fake or Real—Sugars and Fats

Fake or Real—Sugars and Fats
Lecture 32—Transcript

Greetings, and welcome back. In this lecture, I'm going to start out by telling you a story of a little girl that I was working with, who had diabetes, but came to see me for something that was unrelated to her diabetes. She came in and her mom was doing a really great job of managing her diet and her insulin. The problem was the little girl had lots of gas and a lot of diarrhea, so we were exploring all kinds of different dietary strategies. I will admit to you I tried a lot of things until one day she came in and she was chewing gum. I asked her, can I take a look at the kind of gum you're chewing? And she showed it to me, and it was a sugar-free gum made with sorbitol.

Sorbitol is an example of a sugar alcohol, and one of the side effects of too much sorbitol is gas and diarrhea. So although we were looking in a lot of the wrong directions, it was as simple as the gum she was chewing. She just happened to be one of those individuals who is unbelievably sensitive to the effects of sorbitol.

Up to 9 out of 10 American consumers buy or consume products that are low in calories. These products include things such as products that are sugar-free and reduced-fat. They can be beverages or foods. There are numerous products on the market that are made with artificial sweeteners, fat replacers, and other additives. Sometimes it's difficult to determine if what we are eating is real or fake. This lecture will explore the different types of sweeteners and fat replacers used in products from a nutrition perspective, and how they're produced, how they're manufactured. Are they safe? Oftentimes, this is a real concern for American consumers. If you look on the Internet, you can find that sugar replacers are linked with multiple chronic diseases. But is that true or false? What's the proper use of these nutritional replacers?

Let's start out by taking a look at sweeteners. Why are sweeteners a logical place to start? Well, if we're all being honest, we all love sweet foods. Sweetness offers a pleasurable addition to meals and snacks. I always joke that my favorite food in the world is chocolate, and I'll tease my graduate students that when I'm 90, please do not give me any more broccoli. Just give me dark chocolate. Sensitivity to preference levels for sweetness differs from individual to individual. So you may have someone in your family who really doesn't like very sweet foods. It's distasteful to them, but they really prefer things that are salty or crisp.

The preference for sweetness varies by genetics, exposure during early childhood, and whether you are fed or fasted. Another way of thinking about this is, are you full or hungry? Certainly, some people believe that if you have an addictive type of personality, you can actually have a semi-addiction to sugar. Now, I want you to think about this for a second. If you're chronically hungry, you skip breakfast, you skip lunch, most people are going to choose something sweet because it physically makes them feel better. That's not an addiction. That's physiology.

During adolescence, the average intake of sugar is the highest, and for most of us, as we age, this declines. Men in the range of 19 to 50 are in the top category of additional sugar intake, and this refers to sugars added to the foods, not the sugars that are naturally in foods, like milk and fruit. Nearly a third of the extra sugars we consume are from sugar-sweetened soft drinks. Pause and think about this for a second. Think about previous lectures, when we've talked about what's happened with portion sizes. So when Americans are scratching their head and asking, "why am I becoming overweight?" keep in mind this number. Nearly a third of the extra sugars that you consume, or family members consume, come from sugar-sweetened soft drinks.

Additionally, if you're trying to make a dietary change to promote body fat loss, this would be a good place to start. In the United States, most of these sugar-sweetened beverages are actually sweetened with a sugar high-fructose corn syrup. Well, let's start out by taking a look at nutritive sweeteners. What is that definition?

By definition, a nutritive sweetener is something that's sweet tasting, but it also has to have energy associated with it. These are compounds that are generally regarded as safe (GRAS). That GRAS means that the sweetener has been in the food supply for a long period of time, and there's no additional testing needed by the FDA. The common ones that you are familiar with are sucrose, which is table sugar, fructose, which is oftentimes in sugar-sweetened beverages, maple syrups, things such as that. And so again, sucrose is going to have four calories a gram and it's made from sugar cane or sugar beets.

What about fructose as a sweetener? Fructose as a sweetener also has four calories per gram. Again, it's present in fruit and can be added to beverages, such as high-fructose corn syrup. And again, we've talked about this in our lecture on carbohydrates. It's been seen in more and more products on the shelf than products with sucrose for a couple of reasons. It has a higher sweetening power. It is cheaper, and so that's going to be a major consideration. It also has what are called "better functional properties," like flavor, color, and stability. So if I'm a manufacturer and I want to have a product with a longer shelf life, I'm probably going to use a high-fructose corn syrup.

What about digestion and absorption? These are usually easily digestible, unless you have what is called an "inborn error of metabolism," such as galactosemia or inherited fructose intolerance, and you would know that. Our metabolism cannot distinguish which sugars are found naturally in food to those which are added to food. The difference, however, is there's oftentimes more added to food than in a natural product. No matter what the source, we absorb, digest, and metabolize fructose in the same way, whether the fructose again was in the fresh fruit or whether it was added to fruit drinks.

We enter this world of sugar alcohols. They actually are nutritive sweeteners, meaning they are sweet and they have energy. You can tell the difference because almost all the time, they end in the suffix "ol." These are generally regarded as safe food additives. They are often found in baked goods, candy, chewing gum, like my little girl, jams, and jellies. So again, a little bit of caution here. Say for example, you're really trying to buy a loved one a great valentine's present, so you go into the candy store and you say, "I know what I'm going to do. I'm going to buy sugar-free chocolate." Well, I'm going to tell you please don't ever buy that for me because I probably would eat more of that than I needed to have, and those sugar alcohols, again, can cause gas, cramping, bloating, and diarrhea. Again, keep in mind that you might recognize some of these names when you look at the label: manitol, sorbitol, xylitol, maltitol, and then hydrogenated starch. That's probably the exception to our "ol" rule.

Although not universally true, these sugar alcohols usually, again, end in that suffix "ol." Foods with these sweeteners can be labeled as "sugar-free." You may think, well, wait a minute, though. They have calories, don't they? Yes, they do, but they are technically sugar-free. Sugar implies, in general, sucrose or fructose, and again, they're replacing sugar in that food. They provide less energy than the traditional sugars, but if we're going to give them a fair shot here, they also have some other health benefit. If I'm using a sugar alcohol, it actually has a reduced glycemic response because it's incompletely absorbed, so what does that mean?

It means that if we're comparing it to regular table sugar, it's not going to raise your blood sugar as high as regular table sugar would. Because it doesn't have, again, the same biological capabilities of table sugar, it actually has a reduced dental caries risk. So again, dentists are oftentimes happier with sugar-free gums. There's also some suggestion that these sugar alcohols may have a prebiotic effect. Remember, a prebiotic is food for the healthy bacteria that lives in your gut. It hasn't been thoroughly explored, but think about this for a second. If something ends up in my large intestine, it can become food for the healthy bacteria, and again, some of the fermentation products may actually confer some of the health benefits.

What about the absorption and digestion of these foods? This is where they can become friendly or unfriendly. They are absorbed by passive diffusion, meaning these sugar alcohols are absorbed without any transport mechanism. So they kind of passively get into the system. And they are absorbed from the intestine incompletely and slowly. Now, depending on whose research you like to read, more than 20 grams a day of manitol or more than 50 grams of sorbitol, can result in diarrhea, but just like my little girl that I was taking care of, she was consuming around 5 grams of sorbitol per day, and had really pretty extensive GI complications from that. So again, although the research may suggest there's a dose-related response, we are not all identical twins and we may respond differently, just like my little girl.

What about this category of nonnutritive sweeteners? What does that mean? Well, the definition is they still provide a sweet taste, but without energy. That is, they don't have any calories. Five currently have FDA approval, and again, this is oftentimes a moving target. Sometimes there's a sweetener on the market. It leaves, it comes back. By the way, a lot of these products are not available in every store or every region in the country, so you might not be familiar with all of them. Sometimes you might find one in the deep South that's not sold in the Northeast. So let's go through a few of them.

Acesulfame-K is sold as Sunett, Sweet & Safe, and Sweet One, and this is acesulfame-K. Aspartame, which is the one that you might be the most familiar with, is NutraSweet and aspartame in food is marketed as NutraSweet. It is the same compound as Equal. Equal is oftentimes in a little blue pack and it is the tabletop version, but it is the same chemical. What is aspartame because this is going to become important? Aspartame is something called a "dipeptide." Remember, an amino acid is a protein. It's two amino acids that together are sweet. Apart, they are not. We also have a product called "neotame." You also might be familiar with saccharin, which is marketed as Sweet'N Low, Sweet Twin, Necta Sweet, and oftentimes, again, it's the pink packet. If we're talking about colors, now we have sucralose or Splenda, and that's oftentimes the yellow pack.

They all have many similar properties. They are anywhere between 160 to many hundreds of times sweeter than sugar. Neotame, in fact, is several thousand times sweeter than sugar. I want you to think about this. If you're trying to substitute it in a recipe, that's going to be a difficult equation. One of the things that sugar does in a recipe is provide bulk, it provides substance, and it holds water, so it makes food moist or tender. So a cake, for example, that is made with saccharin is not going to have the same kind of physical properties as a cake made with sugar. In fact, it's not going to brown. It's going to be less dense and it's going to be more dry. So again, it may have an increased sweetness, but it's not going to provide all the same physical properties as sugar.

They are all noncariogenic, meaning they do not cause cavities. Aspartame or NutraSweet generates a limited glycemic response, but acesulfame-K, neotame, saccharin, and sucralose generate no glycemic reaction. So why would aspartame cause a slight rise in blood sugar when the other ones wouldn't? This is because aspartame is made from protein, and protein will elicit some glycemic response. Now, in terms of using these products, heating doesn't reduce the sweetening power of acesulfame-K, neotame, saccharin, or sucralose, although prolonged heat may cause a loss of sweetness with aspartame.

Here's a little scientific experiment that you can do with your children or grandchildren to talk about NutraSweet and aspartame and the effects on heat. Get a packet of sugar-free hot cocoa and pour really hot water on it, and let it sit for 45 minutes. It's going to lose its sweetening power the longer it stays in contact with the heat. Those two little amino acids that are sweet when they're together, they break apart in the presence of heat and they're not sweet independent of that. So maybe sometime you might have bought a diet soft drink and you open it up and it really doesn't have any flavor. You think, what's the problem with this? Generally, what's happened is the NutraSweet has broken apart and it's lost its sweetening power. So that probably means that diet soft drink was stored in a warehouse a little bit longer than it should have been, and it broke down due to high heat.

What about saccharin? Well, there's a little bit of a history and an interesting story about saccharin. At one point in time, the FDA almost put it on its most wanted list because it had the potential for carcinogens. Now, not cariogenic, but carcinogens. It had a carcinogen list on the label, and the label listed this, "The use of this product might be hazardous to your health. This product contains saccharin, which has been determined to cause cancer in laboratory animals." But again, let's back up here. The amount of saccharin that was used in these animals to induce bladder cancer, because that's the type of cancer that was developed, was significantly more. It would require you as a consumer to consume hundreds of cans of a diet soft drink a day. That's not realistic, so was there science saying saccharin could cause cancer in laboratory animals? The science said yes, but the amount was impracticable. So in 2000, saccharin had that removed from its label.

These nonnutritive sweeteners may be beneficial in managing diabetes and weight control, in addition to other chronic diseases, as well as preventing cavities. Now, what about sweetener use in health? Here, we're going to take a look at both nutritive and nonnutritive sweeteners. We have very little evidence of detrimental long-term effects on overall health of either nutritive or nonnutritive sweeteners. Now, if I'm raising caution here, I would say that caution should be taken during childhood and pregnancy to avoid excessive amounts of the nonnutritive sweeteners. A lot of the nonnutritive sweeteners haven't been studied in these vulnerable populations, and that should make sense to you why that wouldn't happen. We're not going to expose a pregnant woman to 1000 times the amount of normal sucralose that she should take in. We're not going to do that, so laboratory animals become our models, and again, we have to take caution because oftentimes interpreting laboratory animal data to human data doesn't always work.

The Institute of Medicine say that no more than 25% of calories consumed should be comprised of added sugars, and again, remember, those added sugars are going to be sugars that are in soft drinks, etc. More than that, the dietary quality may be reduced. So again, we have to kind of pause here and think, nutritive sweeteners, sugars that are added in our food supply, can crowd out nutrition. Nonnutritive sweeteners haven't been studied for a long enough period of time, particularly in vulnerable populations, to say that they get out of jail free or get a pass-go card.

What do we know about too much sugar in the diet, though? Too much sugar in the diet may cause the person to decrease consumption of essential vitamins and minerals needed by the body to function. Certainly, excess sugar, along with excess calories, can contribute to obesity. High intakes of sugar-sweetened drinks and foods are associated with an increase in overweight and obesity in children and adults. But keep in mind that if I were to consume a high intake of fat or a high intake of protein, anything in excess beyond my needs can contribute to obesity.

Nonnutritive sweeteners have the potential, and that's a key take-home message here, to reduce the calorie intake. They can save up to 16 calories a teaspoon per sweetening power. The average 12-ounce soft drink, which is now honestly being replaced by the 20-ounce bottles, contains about 150 calories of sugar. If two sodas are consumed each day above your needed calorie level, you can gain 30 pounds in a year. Think about that for a second. You think, I'm not eating that much. How many people ask the question, I wonder if my weight's related to how much I'm actually drinking, and what kind of beverages I'm choosing? So you think, okay, well, I'm not going to drink soda. I'll just drink sweet tea. No, you can't do that either because, again, it's the sugar in the sweet tea. It's not something pathological about the soft drink itself, it's the sugar.

What about diabetes? Are there instances where diabetics might be better off choosing one sweetener versus the other? Due to their incomplete absorption, sugar alcohols cause a lower glycemic response than glucose, fructose, and sucrose. So what does that mean? If a diabetic has a higher blood sugar to begin with, if I can blunt some of that blood sugar rise and still have a sweet product, that might be a good thing. Diabetics may use nonnutritive sweeteners, again, because they don't raise your blood sugar. They don't make your blood sugar more difficult to control.

The science will also say that in a diabetic population, nutritive sweeteners, ones with sugar, ones that have calories in them, should not be completely restricted, but they have to be monitored through proper glucose monitoring. So again, if it's your birthday and you have diabetes and you want a small piece of cake, you may have to get rid of something else that's starchy on your plate to have that small amount of cake with the sugar in it. Again, a saccharin-sweetened birthday cake is probably not going to be something that most of us would enjoy.

Additionally, for those with type 2 diabetes, these nonnutritive sweeteners can aid in weight control. Remember, in the lecture on diabetes, type 2 diabetes is related to obesity, and so if I can reduce the amount of weight that you carry as body fat, I can reduce the likelihood of you developing diabetes. Now, this is where it gets a little bit frightening for consumers. We have to explore a little bit about nutritive and nonnutritive sweeteners and cancer.

According to recent studies in publications, no relationship has been established between the risk of common cancers or cancerous tumors and saccharin, NutraSweet, and other sweeteners. According to recent publications, the potential of artificial sweeteners to cause cancer seems to be insignificant. Now, I will tell you, if you type in "NutraSweet and cancer" in an Internet search, or "Splenda and cancer," you're going to find a lot of websites pop up that are claiming, "I drank Diet Coke and now I have cancer." The challenge with that is the science isn't going to support that, and again, I'm not saying an individual person didn't develop cancer. However, you can't make this quantum leap that everyone who drinks a diet soft drink is going to develop cancer. So again, there's really not a link to nonnutritive sweeteners and cancer development.

We're moving on to fat replacers, and we have to take a look at a few facts here first. Approximately 10% to 15% of all new food products are labeled "Reduced in fat." It's at the top of the list of consumer nutrition concerns. Nutrition concerns of consumers are, Can I lower my fat? Many processed foods, such as meats and cheeses, butter, yogurt, baked goods, and muffins contain fat replacers. These fat replacers must be able to copy some or all of the functional properties of fat in a fat-modified food.

What are the types of fat replacers? These replacers try to imitate the mouth feel of fat being kind of rich and creamy. Most of the fat replacers are going to be classified into three different groups: carbohydrate-based, protein-based, or lipid-based or lipid-modified. You might have heard of some of these, but most of these are used exclusively by manufacturers, so you're not going to be able to go out and buy them necessarily off the shelf.

Let's take a look at the carbohydrate-based fat replacers. Most of the fat replacers are based on carbohydrates. They absorb water, and they can form gels that simulate a texture similar to fat. Sometimes they're used in baked goods and are not, again, routinely available for sale as is. They are oftentimes mixed with water, so they usually provide one to two calories per gram, and they're certainly not appropriate for fried foods. So what are some of these examples? Examples might include fibers, gums, and again, if you're looking at say, for example, a fat-reduced salad dressing, you are going to see one of these words: xanthan, guar, locust bean, alginates. These are all going to be found in diet or reduced-fat salad dressings.

Keep in mind for a second here, if I take all the fat out of a salad dressing and I'm putting in a thickening agent like a gum, my salad dressing really isn't going to pour. It's not going to pour out of a bottle. It might glump out of a bottle because it's binding all the water that's in the salad dressing, and again, it reduces some of its ability to pour. Certainly, dextrins and cellulose, starches and maltodextrins are also going to be used in many of the reduced-fat products. They can contain more than half of the calories of fat, but they also might be higher in sugar.

Let's put on our manufacturer hat for a second. I'm trying to make a product that you like and something that you're going to buy and enjoy and buy again. So you buy a salad dressing and it's Italian and you're looking at the Italian salad dressing bottle. Instead of all your spices kind of floating to the bottle, they're now all suspended in this gel mixture. It clumps on the food. The likelihood is you might not want to buy that again, but if it tastes acceptable, you might. So what manufacturers oftentimes are going to do is they're going to add sugar back to those foods to make it taste a little bit different because you might not like the texture changes that you're seeing.

Fruits can be used as a fat replacer because they have natural fibers, they have pectins and sugars. So think about when your grandmother makes jelly. One of the things that she's going to put in there, or maybe you're the one making jelly, we're going to put in there a product called "Sure-Jell," which is pectin. It holds the juices and now makes that juice essentially spreadable. So examples of fat replacers are things like dried fruits, plums, figs, raisins, applesauce, and bananas. I will tell you, I modify recipes and reduce the fat by using my own natural fat replacers. I'll use applesauce. I've even actually used pumpkin to replace fat in recipes, provided that it's a comparable taste.

Along with the fat replacers, we also have protein-based ones. These are milk, oftentimes whey protein, and remember, whey comes from milk. Remember your nursery rhyme. Little Miss Muffet sat on her tuffet, eating her curds and whey. So whey protein is oftentimes going to be one of the protein-based fat replacers. Egg proteins, again, can be used in the usual source. Again, they're not appropriate for use in fried foods, but they're in many dairy products. Again, also an addition to soups, sauces, creamers, reduced fat butters, sour cream, yogurt, and mayonnaise. You can also see them in ice creams.

Isolated soy protein has been used in some foods as well. A great example of a protein-based fat reducer is something called "Simplesse." It's made from whey or from egg white, and it's through a process called "microparticulation." What they actually do is they take the whey protein or the egg white protein and they incorporate a lot of air, and they give it a mouth feel like fat. So again, I guess you'd call it probably a modification of science to take this protein, whip it with air and give it a product that has a creamy mouth feel. Because it's made from a regular food, it has a GRAS certification, generally regarded as safe. But it would make sense that you can't use it when you bake or when you fry because if I heat up that protein, I'm going to change the way that it looks. Think about a raw egg versus a cooked egg. You're not going to be able to use that in a baking process.

There's modified whey protein concentrate, and again, this whey protein concentrate is going to simulate the mouth feel. An example would be Dairy-Lo. Again, you can't buy that off the shelf, but it's oftentimes used in, let's say, reduced-fat ice creams.

Lipid-based. Now, again, you're thinking, why would I substitute a fat with a fat? Chemical changes can modify this fat so that it will inhibit the absorption or shorten the chain of the length of the fatty acids that produces this lipid-based fat replacer. A great example is a product called "Benefat," and that's actually the commercial name of the product. The generic name is "salatrim." Instead of the nine calories a gram that fat has, it has five calories per gram. It consists of short-chain fatty acids, combined with one long-chain fatty acid that's only partially absorbed. So it's still a fat, but it's been chemically modified so the absorption is somewhat impaired. It's used for foods with low moisture content, such as candies or chocolate chips.

The problem is no warning regarding the side effects was noted by Nabisco, the primary manufacturer, yet some consumers experience nausea, prompting some concerns from public interest groups. Now, why would that be? Again, think of that partially absorbed fat. If it's partially absorbed, that means it's not all absorbed, and again, depending on how fussy your gut is, your gut may not be able to tolerate that partially digested or modified fat.

What about fat extenders? Fat extenders generally have some water associated with it, and a commercial product is something called "Veri-Lo." The calories can be reduced by diluting the fat with water in the form of an oil and water emulsion. I'm sure that you've seen this at the grocery store. If you get a diet margarine, a lot of the diet margarines that are on the market basically have water added to them. So it gives the volume of fat, it spreads on your toast very nicely, but it doesn't have the same amount of calories because in part, what that margarine has is water. So if you ever mistakenly take that margarine and put in a pan to, for example, scramble an egg, all of a sudden, the oil and water separate and you've got a watery mess in your pan. What they've done is they've given the volume of fat, just not the calories of fat.

Fat extenders can reduce the amount of fat in salad dressings, for example, by as much as 70%, and in margarines maybe up to 50%. Lipid analogs have many characteristics of fat, but have a different digestibility and nutritional value. Probably the one that got the most press in the market was a product called "Olean," which essentially is the same compound as Olestra. This gained approval from the FDA in 1996. I remember when the press release came out, saying that this was going to be the wonder fat replacer. It's made from sugar and vegetable oil in a process where a three-carbon glycerol molecule in the oil is replaced with sugar and six to eight fatty acids attached.

I'm going to ask you this question. How delicious does that sound? Does that sound like something that you'd want to put on your dinner table at Thanksgiving? I'm thinking no. This molecule is so large that when it moves through the digestive tract, enzymes don't have the time or the ability to digest the fatty acids. So this was a product that was used in snack foods, for example, frying potato chips. This was really one of the first examples of a fat replacer that could tolerate high heat. There were some problems with this, though. It reduces the absorption of vitamin A and vitamin E. Why would that be the case?

If you remember on your vitamin lecture, vitamin A and vitamin E are fat-soluble vitamins, and so if I'm malabsorbing some fat, if the fat's going in and out without being digested, it's going to drag along those fat-soluble compounds along with it. It can also reduce the valuable carotenoids that are in carrots and cantaloupe and some of the other wonderful foods that I always encourage you to eat. Too much Olestra can cause diarrhea, cramps, and gas. Probably the most popular product that had Olestra in it was WOW potato chips. I am unbelievably sensitive to the effects of Olestra, and I can't have two or three chips without my stomach trying to talk to me and saying, "Roberta, that's probably not a really good idea."

What about the safety of these fat replacers? If the substance is labeled as GRAS, then the FDA supplies the evidence that the fat replacer is safe to use in food. So again, if it's going to be a whey protein, you have whey protein in milk, and so no additional testing needs to be made. But keep in mind that concerns have been associated with the excess use of these fat extenders. One is going to be Olestra and the other one is a compound called "polydextrose," which is a derivative of glucose, that provides bulk. Again, it is oftentimes used as a fat replacer in ice cream. Again, both of these have the ability to cause some degree of stomach upset.

These products have been shown in sensitive individuals to have a laxative effect, resulting in fatty and leaky stools, and the subsequent loss of fat-soluble vitamins. Unfortunately, in my clinical practice, I have seen individuals who were eating WOW potato chips and really had a difficult time making it to the restroom before they really had oily diarrhea. Overall, however, most fat substitutes have shown no known health risks.

Fat replacers and health. What are we going to do about this? If it's used in an overall diet plan that promotes the use of healthy fats and a variety of low-fat products, then a balanced calorie intake can be achieved. Although low-fat products seem to reduce calorie intake, if you consume too many of these products, you'll gain weight. Keep in mind calories in versus calories out still matter. I remember, again, when some of the low-fat foods came on the market, Snackwell's cookies, and maybe you bought them yourself. There's actually something that's been reported to be the "Snackwell cookie effect."

What happened was the minute we labeled it "low fat" or "reduced fat," people thought, okay, well, I can eat as many as I want because it has less calories than a regular cookie. That's where I'm going to say they missed the boat and didn't read the label. Depending on the type of cookie that you would buy, you could get just as many calories in a Snackwell cookie as you could a regular one. Keep in mind what a manufacturer does. If they take out the fat, they want you to enjoy the product, so oftentimes, what they're going to do is put more sugar back in. There is no magic fat replacer that will help to achieve a drastic weight loss, and I think oftentimes, people look at fat replacers or sugar replacers as the magic bullet.

Frequently asked question. I know I can use applesauce as a replacer in some baked goods. Bottom line is how do I use these products? I'm going to tell you that you can use the fruit purees, applesauce, pumpkin, prune, to replace about 50% of the oil that is used in that product. So in my great pumpkin cake recipe, actually I use 50% oil and 50% pumpkin. I have an unbelievably moist cake and it's absolutely delicious. You can reduce the fat in your foods, but having fat-free foods is difficult to obtain.

Thank you very much.

Creating Your Own Personal Nutrition Plan
Lecture 33

What we're going to do is develop a step-by-step road map to a better eating plan ... to help you to be able to review your health history, evaluate your weight, your body mass index, your health status, medications, and to design a basic plan.

Using a nutrition assessment process, you will be able to review your health history; evaluate your weight, body mass index, and medications; and design a basic plan. Keep in mind, this step-by-step guide does not replace advice from your physician or dietitian. Rather, it is intended to personalize the nutrition information you have learned.

We are going to develop a road map to a better eating plan. There are 4 basic assessments—A: anthropometric; B: biochemical; C: clinical; and D: dietary. Anthropometric measurements are body measurements. First, measure your height and weight. Then calculate your body mass index by take your weight in pounds, multiply it by 703, and divide that by your height in inches squared. A body mass index of greater than 25 is considered overweight, 30 or greater is obese, and less than 19.8 is underweight.

Next measure your waist circumference. If it's greater than 35 inches for a woman or greater than 40 inches for a man that means you are likely to develop prediabetes, or metabolic syndrome. If you are able to measure your body composition in a BOD POD, your body fat percentage should be less than 30% for women or less than 20% for men.

For a biochemical assessment, have a physician perform blood work for you. Then look at your cholesterol; your iron status: hematocrit, hemoglobin, and ferritin; and your mean corpuscular volume (MCV). Small red blood cells indicate possible iron deficiency. Large red blood cells mean that you might have B_{12} or folic acid deficiency.

Ask to have your vitamin D status checked. Urinalysis results indicate whether you have sugar or ketones in your urine. It can also indicate the urine concentration: High urine specific gravity indicates dehydration.

Clinical assessment includes any chronic illnesses or medications. Chronic illnesses often require dietary modifications. Medications can cause significant interactions and alter nutritional status.

Your dietary assessment is where you have to be very realistic. Remember, "Progress, not perfection." Half of your plate should be fruits and vegetables, one-fourth should be lean protein, and one-fourth should be whole grains. Alcohol and other liquids can make a big difference in your overall nutrition assessment plan.

To calculate calorie needs, first calculate your ideal body weight using the Hamwi equation (see Table 19) and multiply it by 10 to get your basal metabolic rate. To that, add up to 30% more calories if you are sedentary, 50% if you are moderately active, and 100% if you are active.

Ideal protein intake is 0.8 g per kilogram of your ideal body weight. (To convert pounds to kilograms, divide by 2.2.)

The goals of a nutrition assessment are to provide a baseline of nutritional needs, tolerances, limitations, and the ability to calculate basic nutrition needs. For example, we have a woman who is 5′4″ and weighs 180 pounds. Her ideal body weight is 120, so she needs to lose about 60 pounds. She is sedentary and has high blood pressure. The calorie needs to maintain her ideal body weight are 1500 to 1600 calories per day. She needs to measure her waist circumference for her prediabetes risk; walk 3 miles a day to burn 300 calories so that her diet will not have to be as restricted; use the DASH diet to control her blood pressure; and review her medications with her pharmacist.

Another example is a moderately active man who is 5′8″ and weighs 200 pounds. He has a 44″ waist and is prediabetic. Being moderately active, he needs to eat about 2300 calories to maintain his current weight. To lose weight, he needs to exercise for 1 hour, 5 days a week, and reduce his energy intake. Because of his waist circumference, a Mediterranean diet plan would be a good fit. He might want to consult a registered dietician and review his medications with his pharmacist.

Let's review some frequently asked questions. How can I know if my family makes poor nutrition choices? Become a fruit and vegetable detective. Help them to prechoose their food; look for fruits and vegetables on the menu.

I work very long hours; how can I incorporate a good nutrition plan? You should plan your food for the week in advance; good nutrition does not just happen!

Portion sizes are so small; won't I be hungry all the time following a nutrition plan? No, your calorie needs might be high enough that you would need multiple servings at a meal.

Do children have special nutrition plan needs? Children need more calories than adults per pound of body weight.

Table 19. Sample nutrition plan

What to calculate	How to calculate it	Results	Goals
	Anthropometric assessment		
Height	Measure in inches.		
Weight	Measure in pounds.	_____	_____
Ideal body weight	Use the Hamwi equation. For women: Allocate 100 lb for the first 5 ft and add 5 lb for each inch over 5 ft. For men: Allocate 106 lb for the first 5 ft and add 6 lb for each inch over 5 ft.	_____	_____

225

Body mass index	Multiply your weight in pounds by 703; divide this by your height in inches squared.	_____ _____
Waist circumference	Measure at belly button level in inches.	_____ _____
Body fat composition	Use BOD POD or underwater weighing.	_____ _____
	Biochemical assessment	
Pertinent blood test results	Make sure the blood work checks for cholesterol; iron status including hematocrit, hemoglobin, and ferritin; mean corpuscular volume; and vitamin D status.	_____ _____
Pertinent urinalysis results	Make sure the urinalysis checks for sugar, ketones, and urine specific gravity.	_____ _____
	Clinical assessment	
Chronic illnesses	List all chronic illnesses.	_____ _____
Medications (prescription and over the counter)	List all medicines.	_____ _____
Supplements (vitamins, minerals, herbal therapy)	List all supplements.	

Dietary assessment

(Results of food and exercise diary over 2 weeks)

Ideal caloric intake	Take your ideal body weight from above and multiply it by 10 to get your basal metabolic rate. To that, add up to 30% more calories if you are sedentary, 50% if moderately active, and 100% if active.	_____	_____
Actual caloric intake	Keep a daily food diary, consulting sources such as food labels or CalorieKing.com. Remember to verify portion sizes and the balance and quality of carbohydrates, proteins, and fats.	_____	_____
Alcohol and other beverage intake	Using nutrition labels, factor this into caloric average per day or week.		
Exercise	Calculate average calories burned per day or week; use a fitness log, such as on FitDay.com.	_____	_____

Note: lb = pound; ft = foot. ∎

Suggested Reading

Brown, J., *Nutrition Now*, units 29–31.

McArdle, Katch, and Katch, *Exercise Physiology*, chap. 28.

Questions to Consider

1. What are your ABCD assessment results?

2. What is your personal nutrition plan?

Creating Your Own Personal Nutrition Plan
Lecture 33—Transcript

Greetings, and welcome back. I'm going to tell you a story about a woman that I was working with who had gastric bypass. And she decided that, as part of her wellness plan, she was going to start running marathons. And she came to see me because she was really having some significant gastrointestinal upset. So using the nutrition assessment process, I was able to help her to narrow down the fact that given the fact she'd had gastric bypass, we were going to have to change the type and amount of carbohydrate.

In this lecture, what we're going to do is develop a step-by-step road map to a better eating plan. We are going to use the nutrition assessment process, just like I did with my client, to help you to be able to review your health history, evaluate your weight, your body mass index, your health status, medications, and to design a basic plan. Now, keep in mind this step-by-step guide does not replace advice from your physician or dietician. In your guidebook, you can create your own personal nutrition plan and set your goals. Keep in mind here that our aim is to help you to personalize the nutrition information you have learned, and focus in on progress, not perfection.

What is the nutrition assessment process? It is a process to help you to determine your own nutritional needs and your goals. There are four basic components to the nutrition assessment process, and it's ABCD. Anthropometrics. What does that mean? "Anthropometrics" means measuring the body, so any measurement that you would have would be considered an anthropometric measure. Biochemical or blood or in urine work. So if you have that handy, if you've had a recent physical and you have those numbers handy, that would be the biochemical portion of the nutrition assessment process.

Clinical. What kind of chronic illnesses do you have? What kind of medications do you take on a daily basis? Now, keep in mind when we're talking about medications, it could be things like aspirin. It could be things like an herbal medication that you've tried. What about your multivitamin? Are you taking some vitamin D? So that's an important consideration of this nutrition assessment process. We're also looking at a dietary analysis. What do you eat on a regular basis? Again, keep in mind the nutrition assessment process is designed to help you to set some goals and measure the progress of those goals as change over time.

Now let's explore anthropometric measurements. What is it? Again, it's a body measurement. What are the common ones? Well, first and foremost, it's your height, but you have to measure it. Don't guess and don't rely on your memory. Men tend to overestimate height. For the longest time, I was telling people that I was 5 feet 5 inches, and when I actually measured myself, I'm 5 feet 4(1/2) inches, so I had to take that away. Your weight. Measure it, and measure it in a consistent fashion. So if you routinely get up and weigh yourself without any clothes on, do that as you weigh yourself because, again, you want to be doing it in a consistent way. Women tend to underestimate their weight, so again, make sure that you're measuring these two very important variables.

From these two numbers, you calculate your body mass index. Body mass index is a way of taking a look at height in relationship to weight, and so here's how you calculate it. You take your weight in pounds times 703 and divide it by height in inches squared. What does body mass index tell us? Well, if you have a BMI of greater than 25, you are considered overweight, and greater than 30 is obese. On the other end of the weight scale, less than 19.8 is underweight. Now, keep in mind that BMI cannot tell you what kind of weight you have. So say, for example, you are in the gym on a regular basis and you're strength training, you may have more lean mass that is going to raise your BMI, but you're really not overfat. You may be overweight, but you're not overfat.

Keep in mind that we want to see where that weight is coming from and if that excess weight confers any disease risk, and so we measure waist circumference. Remember what you're trying to do is measure your waist at about the level of your bellybutton. If you have a waist circumference of greater than 35 inches as a woman, greater than 40 inches as a man, you are more likely to develop prediabetes or metabolic syndrome. So it's where you have your weight. Another way of looking at it is if you're looking in the mirror, is your body type an apple, meaning that you've got more of your body fat in your upper body, or are you a pear and have more of your weight in your lower body?

What about body composition? Body composition really rules the day. Check in your community to see if you have access to what is known as a "BOD POD." What a BOD POD does is actually assess how much of your weight is lean mass, and how much of your weight is actually body fat. Truly, I really prefer this as a means of assessing that BMI in a little bit more depth. Again, remember, if I'm lifting weights, I may have an elevated BMI, but I could have a low body fat. We're trying to lower body fat and raise lean mass. So as a woman, your body fat percentage in a BOD POD should be less than 30%, and less than 20% for men.

Another way of getting this done if you're comfortable in the water is underwater weighing. Both of these measures, the BOD POD and underwater weighing, can give us an assessment, a peek on the inside to say how much of my weight is fat and how much of my weight is lean. Body composition is much better than body weight. Now, some people will ask me, what about body fat scales? Well, body fat scales can be reasonably unreliable because think about this for a second. If I stand on the scale, that scale is going to capture my lower body fat better than my upper body fat because it's running a weak electrical current. So it almost always makes men look leaner because men carry more of their fat in their upper body, and it always makes women appear fatter.

You can get calipers done and many personal trainers will use calipers in a gym. The problem with the calipers is it can get the fat right underneath the skin, but it can't capture the fat that's internal, deep inside, that visceral fat that confers disease risk.

What about biochemical assessment? Keep in mind that you have to have a physician who's going to draw blood work for you. This again, is mostly your blood work. What kinds of things would we be looking for as we craft this nutrition assessment plan? Well, keep in mind we're going to look at cholesterol, and you might remember that from previous lectures. You want to take a look at your iron status, so in typical blood work, you might see a hematocrit and hemoglobin, and that can give you kind of a peek as to whether or not you're anemic.

Another thing that may be on your blood work is something called "ferritin," which is the iron that you store that's available in times of need. Another very valuable piece of data on that blood work is something called "mean corpuscular volume," oftentimes abbreviated on your blood work as "MCV." I would encourage you, when you go to your doctor, to ask for an actual copy of the lab slip so you have this, again, as you're crafting your own plan. The mean corpuscular volume means the size of the red blood cell. If you have small red blood cells, chances are you have an iron deficiency. If your red blood cells are large, it means that you might have a deficiency of B_{12} or folic acid.

This next piece of data, the vitamin D status, you might really have to ask for. Physicians are getting better and better at assessing vitamin D status, but when you go and have a physical, ask to have this done. Now, other than blood, what else can we look at? Well, your urinalysis results can take a look at whether or not you have sugar in your urine. That might be, and I stress the words "might be," an indication that diabetes is on your horizon. Does your urine reveal that you have ketones? Ketones are the breakdown metabolites of fat. It also can give us the urine concentration, and this is known as "urine specific gravity." The higher your urine specific gravity, the more likely you are to be dehydrated. So again, the more concentrated or dark your urine is, the more dehydrated you are, and urine specific gravity is a urine test that physicians perform to see how dry or dehydrated you are.

As we go on to clinical assessment, again, this is what makes you really you. It includes any chronic illnesses that you might have. If you have a chronic illness, say, for example, you have diabetes or you're taking any medications, this is a real key part of the clinical assessment portion of the nutrition assessment process. Chronic illnesses oftentimes require some kind of dietary modification, so it's also going to alter the analysis of your diet. It may cause nutrient holes that might need to be filled or avoided. So say for example, you cannot drink milk. If you don't like it or you don't tolerate it, well, now I've created a possible nutrient hole of calcium and vitamin D that I might have to fill with a supplement or with a different food.

Another example might be diabetes, heart disease, or cancer. What about any kind of gastrointestinal disease that you might have? That might include celiac disease or Crohn's disease. These diseases require significant modification and, oftentimes, pharmaceuticals to help to control the disease process. Medications can cause significant interactions and alter nutritional status, and must be taken into account when crafting a nutritional plan. So these are medications, again, that you would use on a chronic basis, not the fact that you would take something like Motrin for a headache.

The most common nutrient-drug interaction, or one that probably causes Americans the most grief in the long run, is grapefruit juice. Grapefruit juice interacts indirectly with over 50% of the commonly used medications. So you would know grapefruit juice as a very nutritious food. If it's pink grapefruit juice, it's got a little red pigment, a little lycopene in it. You think, this is a great thing to have with my breakfast in the morning. The problem is the juice inhibits an enzyme that degrades some of the drug that you might be taking in your intestinal tract. Without the enzyme, and the enzyme is CYP3A4, more medication reaches the blood than is desired. And about 14% of the population drinks grapefruit juice weekly, so keep in mind there are food and drug interactions out there. And again, the ones that we're more concerned about are going to be the ones that you take chronically.

If we're looking at grapefruit juice, what drugs are affected? Well, medication for epilepsy can be affected, antidepressants, calcium channel blockers that are oftentimes used in heart disease, statin resins, drugs that lower your cholesterol, and the effect can last up to 72 hours after you've had your four ounces of grapefruit juice in the morning.

There are also medications that can cause an increase in blood sugar, and this is so important. Say for example, on your regular physical, if the sugar in your urine was a little high, you might want to make sure that you inform your physician that there may be some medications that you're taking that raise your blood sugar, and again, increase the amount of sugar in your urine. What medications can cause an increase in blood sugar? A classification of drugs called "atypical antipsychotics" can cause an elevation in blood sugar. Niacin is a B vitamin, but when used in high enough doses for cholesterol, it can raise your blood sugar.

Medications can also alter your own individual nutritional status. Metformin, which is a very, very common drug for the treatment of diabetes, can actually decrease vitamin B_{12}. So again, if you are on Metformin, this would cue you in when you go to your physician, ask, have you checked my vitamin B_{12} status? I'm a little bit concerned about this interaction. Keep in mind your pharmacist can be a great partner with this. If you're taking methotrexate for rheumatoid arthritis, that can alter folic acid status, and certainly, over-the-counter medications and herbal medications can also affect nutritional status. A very, very popular herb called "Chinese red yeast extract" can lower cholesterol in a similar fashion as the statin resins. Fish oil can lower triglycerides, and so medications and chronic illnesses really play a big part in the nutrition assessment process.

So what about the "D" in nutritional assessment? Well, the "D" stands for dietary assessment. Now, this is where you have to be very realistic. How does your diet stack up? Again, remember, our goal here is always progress, not perfection. So I will declare openly my favorite food in the world is chocolate, so I have no problem saying, "That might be the thing in my diet that might be a weakness for me." But you can rate your own plate. Fifty percent of your plate should be fruits and vegetables, one-fourth should be some source of lean protein—and remember, a lean protein could be beans, it doesn't have to be meat—and one-fourth should be a whole grain.

There are some great websites out there, and one of my favorite is a website called "Rate Your Plate" by the University of Connecticut's Team Nutrition. It's interactive; it has pull-down menus. It has interactive ways of designing your own plate. It's a wonderful tool. There are also interactive nutrition and physical activity monitoring systems. Again, one of my favorite is something called www.FitDay.com, and it's a website where you log in, you log in your food intake and your exercise to see how you're progressing. So what you're actually doing is evaluating your nutritional status and your progress as you try and make dietary changes.

Keep in mind that dietary changes are difficult for most of us to make because we have habits, we have preferences. So again, keep in mind that we're looking at progress, not perfection. However, the key to understanding any online program is you have to understand portion sizes because any online program is going to ask you, "What was your serving size?" or "What was your portion size?" If your portion size is incorrect, your assessment of calories and protein is also incorrect. So can you eyeball portions? Well, a half a cup is about the size of the palm of your hand. Now, I realize not all of us are the same size, and for a very large man versus a petite woman, the palm of the hand is going to be different, but as a crude estimate, a half a cup is about the size of the palm of your hand. So if you had pasta last night and it covered your plate, you didn't have a half-a-cup portion. That's probably a two-cup portion.

Three ounces of meat is about the size of a deck of cards, and I like that as an analogy because it also gives us depth. An ounce of cheese is about the size of a domino. I want you to think about that for a second. Cheese is a very high-fat protein, about 100 calories per ounce. So if you have six ounces of cheese and crackers, you had 600 calories of cheese. A half a cup of rice or potatoes or ice cream or a sticky or creamy food is about the size of a tennis ball. So if you get out a big cereal bowl and have ice cream at night, you're not having a half-a-cup portion.

What about websites to help you count calories? Well, there is www.calorieking.com and others than can help you to determine the calories in the food you eat. I think that's a really great thing to do because calorieking and a lot of the calorie-counting websites can actually help you to look at fast foods or favorite restaurants that you might frequent as well.

What about alcohol intake? Alcohol and other liquids can oftentimes be overlooked as a source of energy. We tend to remember what we eat, but not so much what we drink. As little as two regular beers per day would add up to 2100 calories per week. If you're trying to lose weight, there's 3500 calories in a pound, so those liquid beverages can make a big deal in your overall nutrition assessment plan.

Can you do a more in-depth analysis of your needs? Let's take a look at calorie needs. First and foremost, we have to calculate ideal body weight, and I'm going to remind you there's an equation out there that we've talked about before called the "Hamwi equation," but let's review it. It allows 100 pounds for the first five feet of height for women, and five pounds for each inch after. Men get a little bit more weight for the first five feet of height. It's 106 pounds for the first five feet, and six pounds for each inch after. The value of this is once you take your ideal body weight, so again, if I'm 5 feet 4 inches, I'm going to round down here, my ideal body weight is 120, and 120 times 10 gives me the calories that are needed for my basal metabolic rate. So that gives me my BMR calories.

To that, I can add up to 30% additional calories if I'm sedentary, 50% if I'm moderate, and 100% if I'm active. The problem is most people confuse being busy with activity. So to be moderately active, for example, I would have to have some activity in my daily life, like being a nurse in a hospital. And then I would have to get regular exercise outside of that. So unfortunately, in our lifestyle today, a pretty high percentage of us actually are sedentary. So again, let's use that example of a woman who's 5 feet 4 inches and moderately active. Her ideal body weight would be 120. And 120 times 10 is 1200. If she's moderately active, she can add up to 50% of those BMR calories, which is 600, and her total energy needs would be 1800 calories. Now, keep in mind, she could be consuming more energy than that, and that slight increase in energy can cause weight gain, maybe not instantly, but over a period of time.

I'll give you an example. If she requires 1800 calories a day, and just eats 1900 calories a day, she'll gain 10 pounds in a year, and quite honestly, that's the way most Americans gain weight. It's what I call the "insidious weight creep." All of a sudden, your clothes are a little bit tight. We blame the manufacturer. It wasn't the manufacturer. We have these increasing calories that are creeping up. Now, what about a man? A man who is 5 feet 10 inches and sedentary, has an ideal body weight is 166, 166 times 10 is 1660. If he's sedentary, he only gets to add 30%, so 30% would give him a total energy need of 2158. Again, remember, if you're trying to lose weight, you have to cut between 500 and 1000 calories per day.

What about if you're underweight and you need to gain weight? Well, it's the reverse. You would add 500 to 1000 calories per day. Now, what about protein intake? Protein intake is a little bit more difficult, so you might want to get out a calculator, a piece of paper, and a pen. It's 0.8 grams per kilogram of ideal body weight. It's not based on what you weigh, but on what you should weigh because again, remember, protein is needed to build and repair lean body mass. So this 120-pound woman, ideal body weight is 120, and to go from pounds to kilos, you divide by 2.2, and that'll give you 54.5 kilos. 54.5 times 0.8 gives her a total protein need, rounded up, of 44 grams of protein per day. Honestly, that's very easy to get in a traditional American diet.

Let's use our male example as well. He's 5 feet 10 inches, ideal body weight is 166. I have to convert that to kilos. I divide by 2.2 and he's 75 kilos. And 75 times 0.8 is 60 grams, and again, very easily met by most dietary plans. An exception to that might be if you're a vegan. So if we're using our deck of cards, 3 ounces of meat the size of a deck of cards is equal to 21 grams of protein. So a serving of meat for our female example is almost half of the protein that she needs per day, and that's, again, very easy to get in an American diet. So most of us, as typical Americans, if you're a carnivore, chances are you over-consume rather than under-consume protein.

What if you have an older person in your life? Are there any tools out there? Or if you're a senior yourself and you're concerned about your dietary requirements, I would encourage you to consult what is called the "DETERMINE questionnaire" on the website of the American Academy of Family Physicians. It's an easy-to-use validated screening tool, designed to determine nutritional risk in older individuals. What it would do is it would ask some questions about diet. It's self-administered. That would be the "D" portion. So for example, it might ask the question, "How many meals do you eat per day?" If you eat two or less meals per day, you're going to increase your nutritional risk. It would ask about weight loss. Have you lost weight in the last six months, not as part of a purposeful weight loss plan? So again, it's a great, validated tool, and again, you can find it on that particular website.

The goals of nutrition assessment are to provide you a baseline requirement of nutritional needs, tolerances, limitations, and the ability to calculate basic nutrition needs. So let's try and pull all this together with an example. We have a woman who is 5 foot 4 inches and she currently weighs 180. So you're thinking in the back of your mind, 180 is probably not her ideal body weight, so let me figure this out. She should weigh 120. That would tell you from the beginning that she's got about 60 pounds to lose. She's sedentary, with high blood pressure. She doesn't drink any alcohol, but she drinks black tea. Calorie needs to maintain her weight would be ideal body weight times 10, 1200. She's sedentary, so we add a third to get somewhere in the range of 1500 to 1600 calories per day. To lose weight and to do an effective nutrition assessment, she would need to do the following.

We would want her to measure her waist circumference to check her risk of prediabetes. With the approval of her physician, we might want her to walk three miles a day to burn about 300 calories. Why is that the case? Her calories are already reasonably low to maintain her weight, and so one of the strategies would be if I can get her to move, I don't have to restrict her food quite as much. So she could walk three miles per day to burn 300 calories. And I would want her to reduce her energy intake by about 200 calories per day to reach the 500 calorie per day goal that we're looking for. Because she's hypertensive, we would want her to include the principles of the DASH diet to help to control her blood pressure—more fruits and vegetables, low-fat dairy. She also is going to need to review her medications with her pharmacist to make sure her high blood pressure medication does not cause her to lose potassium or to cause her blood sugar to be elevated.

So again, that's a quick example of what she could do to say, "I'm going to pull all of this together. I'm going to tie it up in a nice bow and I'm going to have, again, a little bit more of a nutrition action plan." I think the challenge is for most Americans who are sedentary, they're not going to be satisfied with just reducing calories alone because bottom line is you're going to be hungry. The other challenge here, and it's a real challenge, is that most Americans are relatively impatient with weight loss. So if we restrict her by 500 calories a day, she's not going to have a 10 pound per week weight loss. Again, most Americans will say, "I was on a diet for a week, and I only lost a pound." Rather than feel depressed, I would say, "You need to cheer because the chances are you've created a plan that you can live with." Because what we're looking, again, for is progress, not perfection.

Let's come up with an example for a man. He's 5 foot 8 inches, weighs 200 pounds, but he is moderately active. Maybe he has a job as a lineman for a utility company, and he goes out and exercises, plays handball with his buddies a couple of times a week. But that waist circumference—he's gotten out his tape measure. He's got a 44 inch waist and he's been diagnosed as prediabetic. He drinks one beer every single evening and when he actually critically evaluates his diet, he's taking in two teaspoons of sugar in his coffee, and he has three cups a day. The calories he needs to maintain his weight would be about 1540. He's moderately active, so he can add half of that to figure out his total daily calorie intake, at about 2300 calories per day. But to lose weight, he would need to do the following.

Walk or work out at a gym for one hour, five days a week, so maybe I want him to ramp up his activity, and then he would have an additional 400 calorie loss each day, which would total about 2000 calories for the week, and I want him to reduce his energy intake by about 250 calories per day to total a loss of 1750 per week. So 250 calories cut out of a diet really isn't that difficult to do. He could reduce his alcohol intake to maybe one beer per week, and save 900 calories per week. But again, all of us are going to have our own individual preferences. Maybe that's not where he wants to save calories. Maybe there's something else he could do in his diet. For example, maybe he would change from eating red meat to chicken, and save some calories that way.

Another strategy that he could try is to use a sugar substitute in his coffee, which would save 36 calories per cup, three cups per day, every day. He could save 750 calories per week by doing that. Again, because of his waist circumference, we might be looking for a low-fat, low-calorie diet for him, and a Mediterranean diet plan would be a good fit. So when we add up all the numbers, 2000 calories lost here, 1750 here, 900, 750, he would lose about 5400 calories per week and lose weight at about a rate of 1.5 pounds per week. Now, again, he might want to consult a registered dietician to make sure he's on the right path for dealing with his prediabetic condition. He's going to need to review his medications with his pharmacist to avoid food and drug interactions. And ideally, this is the kind of patient I really love to work with because he's on the verge of a disease. If we can prevent that disease from actually manifesting itself, now he's in a wonderful position to prevent diabetes and prevent some of the consequences associated with diabetes.

What about our frequently asked questions? I try to eat right and prepare good meals at home, but it's my children and my husband that eat out at lunch. How can I know if they make poor nutrition choices? Do we have any advice for that? Well, become a fruit and vegetable detective. If you're worried about your children eating well at school, you may want to involve them, for example, in preparing their lunch, or if they eat a school lunch, what you may want to do is actually print off or take a look at the nutrition information online from your school district and help them to pre-choose before they go.

You can also become a fruit and vegetable detective. Almost every type of restaurant, and fast food outlet, has fruits and vegetables, if you look. The problem is when we go into a fast-food restaurant, we don't look at the menu. We oftentimes choose by number, and then we supersize it. So what we're actually going to do is just encourage people if they eat out at a fast-food restaurant not to supersize and avoid sweet liquid calories. In my experience, the average supersize meal is going to be about 2000 calories. Keep that in mind. We just went through all those calculations. You go and have one fast-food meal that you've supersized and that would be more calories that I could eat for the entire day.

Another frequently asked question, "I work very long hours, sometimes 10, 12 hours a day. How can I incorporate a good nutrition plan into such a lifestyle?" Actually, when you're doing your dietary analysis as part of this nutrition assessment process, when you get to diet, critically look at your barriers. We all have them, and so a barrier for someone who works very long hours is they're going to probably need to plan their food, take a little bit of time on a Sunday evening, pack up some food, stock a refrigerator at work with yogurt, fruits, and vegetables. What I usually will say is, "You know what? Good nutrition just doesn't happen. For very busy and active lifestyles, you actually have to put some forethought into it." So again, plan your food, and it's as easy as just packing some extra fruits and vegetables.

Another frequently asked question. "Wow, portion sizes are so much smaller than I thought." This is one of the reasons, and in my experience, one of the driving factors, on how individuals don't assess their diet in a reasonable fashion. Keep in mind that 50 years ago, people ate dessert. They ate fried foods, but the portions were smaller. So the challenge always is, aren't I going to be hungry all the time if I follow any kind of nutrition plan? Well no, not really because your calorie needs might be high enough that you would need multiple servings, for example, of bread at a meal. So you might need more bread and cereal than the half a cup portion. The more calories you need, the greater your portion sizes. But again, a single portion for a starch, for example, like rice is about the size of the palm of your hand.

Another frequently asked question is, can a nutrition plan be used for children? Don't they have special needs that adults don't? Yes, children need more calories than adults per pound of body weight. The challenge is children have a smaller body weight, so calories per pound are higher, but total energy needs are not. Children need a variety of food, and what is unique here is that children usually have increased appetite during growth spurts. Parents and grandparents should not attempt to control children's calories or to count them. But what you can do is stress lean meats, low-fat dairy, and fruits and vegetables. Again, remember, children have this wonderful gift. We're all born with the ability to eat when we're hungry and stop when we're full. Please don't try and aggressively control your children or grandchildren's diet.

Thank you very much.

Exercise and Nutrition—Partners for Life
Lecture 34

Being healthy is not just a matter of what you eat. It's also a matter of being physically active throughout the day.

Many diseases and negative health conditions are related to having an inactive lifestyle and are preventable through routine physical activity and exercise. Exercise has physical health benefits: It reduces the risk of heart disease, hypertension, stroke, colon cancer, and breast cancer; it can help to build bone mass and prevent the bone loss associated with aging; and it can help to reduce the risk of obesity or control obesity and reduce diabetes.

There are also psychological health benefits: It increases feelings of well-being, decreases depression and anxiety, and helps to relieve stress. A better body image improves self-esteem and motivational levels.

The American College of Sports Medicine gives the following guidelines. For 5 days a week, do moderately intensive cardio for 30 minutes a day; or for 3 days a week, do vigorously intensive cardio for 20 minutes a day. For 2 days a week, do 8 to 10 strength training exercises with 8 to 12 repetitions of each exercise.

[Exercise] increases feelings of well-being, decreases depression and anxiety, and helps to relieve stress.

Weight bearing, or resistance, exercise helps build muscles and tone muscle fibers. Overloading the muscle allows it to adapt. There are different types of resistance training. Calisthenics uses your own body weight and no equipment. Fixed or constant resistance provides a constant amount of resistance through a full range of motion. Variable resistance is where the amount of resistance changes through the full range of motion.

Raise the weight in a deliberate and smooth manner. When you get the weight up to the fully contracted position, pause. Slowly shift from the raising to the lowering of the weight. To strengthen your muscles, make your muscles work against a gradually increasing resistance. Then increase the resistance, the number of repetitions or sets, or the intensity. Specificity is another training principle, but for an overall positive effect, you should strengthen all major muscle groups. To determine how much strength training is necessary use the FITT principle: frequency, intensity, time, and type.

Endurance exercise includes aerobic and anaerobic exercise. Aerobic exercise uses the body's ability to deliver oxygen to muscles for physical activity. Some of the benefits include reduced body fat, improved weight control, reduced blood pressure, decreased total cholesterol, improvement in heart and lung function, lowered resting heart rate, and improved glucose tolerance. Aim for a minimum of 3 days a week of aerobic exercise, with no more than 2 days off between sessions.

Anaerobic means without oxygen. This is short-lasting, high-intensity exercise. The benefits include the development of stronger, oftentimes bigger, muscles. For beginners who are not very fit, try interval training to incorporate anaerobic exercise.

Your exercise plan must also include the following. Stretching muscle groups increases flexibility and range of motion. It helps to protect muscles and tissues from injuries or tears. Hydration is important. Dehydration can impair exercise performance and can become life threatening. If you need some nutrition before exercise, consume a meal or a snack; during exercise for more than an hour, consume a sports drink; after exercise, consume adequate fluids and energy. Overall, increase your intake of whole grains, cereals, and legumes. Get 5 or more servings of fruits and vegetables a day. Consume adequate amounts of water throughout the day. It is important to develop a plan that feels right and will last for you.

Let's review some frequently asked questions. Do I have to do my half hour or hour of exercise all at one time? No, you can split it up.

Should I exercise when I am sick? No, you need to take a couple of days off. ∎

Suggested Reading

Mahan and Stump, *Krause's Food, Nutrition, and Diet Therapy*, chap. 25.

McArdle, Katch, and Katch, *Exercise Physiology*, chaps. 3, 7, 23, 29, 32.

Questions to Consider

1. What proof do you have in your life or your family members' lives that exercise is medicine?

2. What is your personal exercise plan?

Exercise and Nutrition—Partners for Life
Lecture 34—Transcript

Hello, and welcome back. I'll start off by telling you a relatively embarrassing story about myself. When I first started at the Houston Texans, I had weight trained my whole entire life, and I was working with the strength coach. I said, "Yeah, I know how to lift weights. I know how to do that." And he started training me, and I describe it as a religious experience because the workouts were hard and intense. But one of the fortunate things that I did was I took a look at what my body composition was before I started weight training, and in my eight years at the Texans, I've gained a documented seven pounds of muscle mass by resistance training. I will tell you, at my age, that's probably one of the most beneficial things that I could do, is to add as much functional lean mass as possible.

The point of this is that being healthy is not just a matter of what you eat. It's also a matter of being physically active throughout the day. This is so important as a public health campaign that it's now part of the food guide pyramid, so if you look at the food guide pyramid, you can watch a little man climbing up the stairs. It's trying to demonstrate the marriage of physical activity and good nutrition as part of an overall wellness plan. Many diseases and detrimental health conditions are related to being inactive. They also can be prevented through routine physical activity and exercise.

In this lecture, we'll discuss the basic components of an exercise program. This has become so important to promote physical activity among Americans that the American College of Sports Medicine has, as a campaign, exercise is medicine. They really want Americans to embrace the concept that sometimes it's lifestyle, nutrition and physical activity, that's going to ward off chronic illness. It may not be another pharmaceutical. So this lecture's also going to take a look at how an average person can implement physical activity into his or her daily lifestyle. I'm going to caution you here, however, that if you have a pre-existing health condition, for example, if you have diabetes, you really want to make sure that you clear this with your primary physician before you implement an exercise program.

Let's take a look or explore some of the benefits of exercise. Physical health benefits: It reduces the risk of certain diseases and disorders, such as heart disease. Studies show that being fit or active was associated with reducing the risk of cardiovascular-related diseases by 50%. Now, think of what that means. I'm also going to suggest to you here that sometimes the benefits of disease prevention are the best in people who go from doing nothing to doing something. So you might say, well, I've not exercised. I'm relatively sedentary. I don't really like physical activity. Some is always going to be better than none, and it's that initial startup where you get a significant benefit from starting a physical activity program.

Exercise can also reduce the risk of hypertension and stroke. What about cancer? Well, one study showed that people who are physically active, men and women, can reduce the risk of colon cancer by 30% to 40%. So again, as we talk about cancer as being a feared diagnosis, wouldn't it be wonderful to include physical activity as part of your wellness portfolio? What about breast cancer? The same study revealed that compared to inactive counterparts, there is a 20% to 30% reduction in relative risk of breast cancer. So again, we know that heart disease and cancer are two major killers of Americans, and now we can link being physically active to the prevention of those diseases.

What about bone disease, osteoporosis? Well, what exercise can do is it helps to build bone mass, and the older you get, it can help to prevent falls and reduce the risk of hip fractures. It can prevent the bone loss associated with aging. So it almost sounds like it's too good to be true, and in this case, it's not. Physical activity is that good. It can also help to reduce your risk of obesity, or control obesity, particularly that excessive abdominal fat that is linked, again, with many chronic diseases.

Diabetes. One lifestyle intervention study found that a minimum of 150 minutes per week, not per day, of exercise was more effective in reducing diabetes than metformin alone. So what does that mean? It means that lifestyle matters in the prevention of chronic illness, as well as the treatment of chronic illness. Beyond the physical, there are psychological health benefits. It increases your feeling of wellbeing. Studies suggest it decreases depression and anxiety. It can help to relieve stress. A better body image improves self esteem and motivational levels. So we've got this wonderful solution to, again, chronic illness.

Exercise helps to control long-term weight. An energy deficit of 500 to 1000 calories per day is necessary to achieve a healthy one to two pound weight loss per week, and that energy deficit is best achieved through a well balanced diet, making some changes that you can live with, and I will always tell my clients, make the dietary changes that are going to become permanent, and increase your physical activity. Consider that when you introduce physical activity, you have a better guarantee that what you're losing is body fat, and not just weight loss. The body needs more energy calories to maintain muscle, so the more muscle mass you have, the higher your calorie needs. So I was relatively excited that my measured metabolic rate went from 1200 calories when I started at the Texans to 1600 calories per day by adding that seven pounds of lean mass.

Keep in mind that as you build muscle, the more muscle mass you have, the bigger your metabolic engine, and the higher your calorie needs at rest. So again, this helps to burn more calories at rest than the average person would. So if our authoritative organization here is the American College of Sports Medicine, what do the experts say? ACSM recommends the following: For five days a week, do moderately intensive cardio for a half an hour a day. What is cardiovascular exercise? It's walking, gardening, not necessarily going to a gym. You can certainly do a lot of cardio activity outside. Or three days a week, do vigorously-intense cardio for 20 minutes a day. And their newest recommendation is two days a week, do 8 to 10 strength training exercises with 8 to 12 repetitions of each exercise.

I actually have a wonderful picture of my daughter's college, and you look at the cardiovascular equipment. All the women are on the treadmill and the elliptical, and all the men are doing weight training. What we need to do is have them cross the great divide and have women strength training and maybe men doing a little bit more work on the elliptical. Now, by "moderately-intense physical activity," we mean working hard enough to start perspiring and increase your heart rate. By "vigorous exercise," we mean that if you're running with a friend, if it's vigorous, little conversation could be exchanged, just a few words. Sometimes that's referred to as the "talk test."

The recommendation for a half an hour, five days per week is for an average healthy adult to maintain general good health and reduce the risk for the chronic diseases that we mentioned. However, if weight loss is your goal, if you're trying to lose weight, or you've lost weight and you want to maintain your weight loss, it may be necessary to do an hour to an hour and a half of physical activity a day for five days a week. So one of the challenges is, as we become more sedentary as a culture, we have more things that are convenient. I remember my mother washing her clothes down in the basement with a hand washing machine, and then walking outside and hanging it up on a clothes line. We have too many conveniences in our modern day society, and we get less and less exercise. So ACSM has addressed this by almost giving you an exercise prescription.

What are the components of exercise? Let's talk about physical fitness and let's define it. The ACSM definition is a state of health measured by strength, endurance, and flexibility. They don't define physical fitness as huge muscles, being ripped, a tiny waistline, or anyone like a bodybuilder with a large amount of muscle mass. What is strength? It's the level of maximum force that the muscles can produce. So I'm going to have you think about that for a second. It's the level of maximum force, so if you're one of these folks that are going to the gym and you're lifting really, really, light weights, that's probably not strength producing exercise.

Endurance is the length of time muscles can perform activities. Flexibility is range of motion. All of those are important. Well, what about muscular strength? Weight bearing or resistance exercise is important in order to build muscles and tone muscle fibers. Unfortunately, as I've mentioned, our current lifestyle doesn't require lifting. Now, I want you to consider what's known as the "overload principle." In order to get stronger, you have to ask the muscle to do more work than it can. Overloading the muscle allows it to adapt. What does that actually mean? I'll give you a quick example.

You're going to do, let's say, a bicep exercise, where you're raising and lowering the weight. If your muscle is capable of lifting 10 pounds, and that's all you ever do, you're not going to get any stronger. You're not going to build strength. Your muscle adapts to that overload. It's now conditioned to that overload, and it technically isn't overloaded any more because the muscle is already accustomed to that. The frequency of strength training should be about two times per week, both upper and lower body. Keep in mind that what you're trying to do is have equal strength. I'm also going to say on both sides of the body because oftentimes what we do is when we strength train, we train the muscles we can see because we're looking in the mirror. We train the muscles we can see, and we forget about our backside.

As you become more conditioned or more trained, the number of days of training can increase. Now, keep in mind that injuries can happen in the weight room, and some sources say the most frequent injury site is the lower back. Consider hiring a trainer to help to develop a program for you, and meet with you on an ongoing basis. A really good strength conditioning professional can modify a program for you, based on your individual needs. Again, a good place to look for that person is at ACSM.org.

Let's talk about some general concepts. Let's talk about the type of resistance training. The types of resistance training can vary, and first is calisthenics. It's using your own body weight in general, without using any equipment. So this would include push-ups, pull-ups, crunches, squats, lunges, and so forth. But let's say, for example, I'm someone who loves doing crunches, and every morning when I get up, I do 25 crunches. Once my muscle adapts to 25 crunches, I've got to do one of two things. I've got to find a way to add weight and maybe what you do is take, let's say, a couple of cans of beans, cross them across your chest when you do your squat because you want to add some additional weight to that squat or that crunch to make sure that you're going to get adequate amounts of overload.

There's also something called "fixed" or "constant resistance," which is exercise that provides a constant amount of resistance through a full range of motion. The most common examples here include the use of free weights, resistance bands, and certain machines. So I have a lot of clients who travel with their resistance bands because they can't honestly bring barbells or dumbbells in their suitcase.

Variable resistance is exercises where the amount of resistance changes through the full range of motion. Some of these are machines that alter the resistance. You might not know it, but the machine is altering the resistance for you, so when you're weaker, it may back off the weight. When you're stronger, it's going to actually add some additional weight for you.

So what about your resistance training plan? How do you put that together? You want to raise the weight in a deliberate and smooth manner. So I'm going to suggest to you that you do not use momentum. So if you've ever been in a weight room, you see individuals take the weight and they swing their hips to get the weight up. You've now incorporated momentum into that lift, and it's not as effective. You've reduced the amount of weight that you're lifting because you've incorporated momentum. So raise the weight in a deliberate and smooth manner.

For a moment, when you get the weight up to its fully contracted position, pause. At this point, the muscle fibers are fully contracted. You've got every muscle fiber engaged, and that's a really good thing in terms of helping you to add some strength. Slowly shift from the raising to the lowering of the weight. And if I could tell you one major tip, it's to really emphasize the lowering of the weight. Half of the benefit comes from raising the weight, and the other half of the benefit comes from lowering the weight. Take more time to lower the weight.

I want you to think about this. When you're raising the weight, you're going against gravity. When you're lowering the weight, you have gravity working in your favor, and so truly, if you want to make the exercise harder, one of the ways you can do this is to take more time. So I actually count. I'll count five seconds up, pause in the contracted position, and then I'll count up to eight while lowering the weight. I will tell you this makes the resistance training exercise much more difficult to do.

Most of the muscular damage is done in this phase, and you might be saying to yourself, I don't want to damage my muscles. But actually, what you're trying to do is cause small little microtears in that muscle, and the muscle's going to have to adapt, get stronger and strengthen those muscle fibers, i.e. toning, or add more muscle fibers. That's exactly what resistance training is designed to do. You also want to go through the full range of motion, not these little half raises that you see people doing in the gym. The full range of motion, okay?

To strengthen your muscles, you must include activities that make your muscles work against a gradually increasing resistance. Again, I cannot over stress the overload principle and how important it is. Keep in mind that it can be achieved by doing the following: Once you're accustomed to it, you increase the resistance. Use a heavier weight. I always say I want to lift the most amount of weight as safely as I can every time I go to the weight room. If that's not a possibility for you, you can increase overload by increasing the number of repetitions of exercises, again, the number of raising and lowering motions, such as a bicep curl.

You can also increase the number of sets that you perform, and a set is a group of repetitions. So instead of doing two sets of 8, you might do two sets of 10, or maybe three sets of 10, and gradually increase that. Increasing the intensity, more work in the same amount of time, so what you're really trying to do is get those muscles to work harder.

Specificity is another training principle. Exercising a certain muscle or muscle group targets and develops that part. For an overall positive effect, we need to strengthen all major muscle groups. The bad news is if you stop training, we see evidence of the reversibility or the detraining principle. Within a few weeks of stopping training, you lose some of the strength that you've built up. So again, when you're designing your exercise program, you think, the American College of Sports Medicine is telling me that I need to do this at least twice a week. That means 52 weeks out of the year. It's not an occasional thing. It's not, maybe I'll do this once a month. This is something that you have to build into your exercise program. Muscles can atrophy without use, and that's what generally happens to people when they age.

How much strength training is necessary? Well, use the FITT principle. What does this mean? It means frequency. How often do you exercise? Again, in accordance with the ACSM guidelines, at least two days a week, 8 to 10 strength training exercises that train each muscle group. So again, you might do biceps, triceps, quads, the front of your leg, and the hamstrings, the back of your leg. Plan for at least one to two days of rest in between because, again, what you're trying to do is make the muscle work really hard, cause some microfiber tears, and then you allow the muscles to heal and go back again.

The second part of the FITT principle is intensity. How hard do you exercise? The training session should be challenging to you. If you're training with a partner who's been training for a while, what's challenging to them and you might be something completely different. I think, oftentimes, when people get exercise religion, what they do is they go into a weight room, they lift too much weight. They're not capable of doing it, and then the next day, they're so sore that they don't want go back and do that. You need to have enough intensity that by the time you're done with your last repetition, your muscle should feel fatigued. I always describe it as I really couldn't do one more. I'm to the point where my muscle is tired enough not to be able to do one more.

A "T" in the FITT principle is time. How long do you exercise? For strength training, this is measured as the number of sets or reps that you do, although the intensity and your form are always important. Give yourself some rest period in between sets. Between 30 to 90 seconds is typical. The other part of the FITT principle, the other "T" is what type of exercises you do. Exercises you do should target every major muscle group. I will tell you, in professional football, most of the major injuries that football players sustain are going to be to their neck and their traps, their upper shoulder muscles. The challenge is our football players must train their neck because they're trying to protect themselves against a catastrophic injury.

Keep in mind that we're talking about all muscle groups. Again, you have to remember to work opposing muscle groups, the front and the back, biceps and triceps, the hamstrings in the back and the quads in the front. You can try this FITT principle for other forms of exercise, besides strength training as well. You can use the FITT principle for endurance. "Endurance exercise" or "aerobic exercise" is defined as the ability to deliver oxygen to muscles, and the capability of muscles to use oxygen for physical activity. "Aerobic" means with oxygen. "Aerobic" also means performing activities that increase the heart rate for a longer period of time. Some of these activities would include jogging, playing basketball, soccer, swimming, low- to moderate-intensity activities that can be sustained for a long period of time.

What are the benefits for aerobic or endurance exercise? Reduced body fat and improved weight control, reduced blood pressure, decreased total cholesterol, improvement in heart and lung function, lowered resting heart rate. Remember, if your heart's beating harder on a regular basis, you may be overworking it, and so again, if I lower my resting heart rate, I can actually get some real beneficial health effects from that. Aerobic or endurance exercise also improves glucose tolerance, so again, if you're that person sitting on the fence of prediabetes, remember that exercise is medicine in this case. What you're really trying to do is prevent diabetes from becoming full blown. It reduces insulin resistance.

How do I know if I'm training aerobically? How do I know if I'm getting all those benefits? One of the things that you can do is to check your pulse rate. Here's what you do. You measure your pulse rate immediately after you're done exercising. Place your fingertip, not your thumb, on your carotid or neck artery, and count the number of pulses you feel in a 10-second period. Multiply this by 6 to determine your heart rate. What should your heart rate be? Maximum heart rate has a prediction equation, so it's not universally true and there are some medications that can alter this, and this is why you always want to check with your physician. Maximum heart rate is predicted to be 220 minus your age. So if I'm 50 years old, my maximum heart rate is 220 minus 50, which is 170 beats per minute.

Beginners should strive for between 40% to 60% of their maximum heart rate, and work up to a higher level. So if our 50 year old is a beginner, her heart rate should be up to 170 beats a minute times 0.6. The heart rate maximum for that individual to train aerobically would be 102 beats per minute. Aerobically fit people, so if you've already been running and jogging, if you're already fit, they should aim for 70% to 85% of their maximum heart rate levels. So our 50 year old, in order to be in the aerobic training zone, has a target heart rate of between 119 and 144 beats per minute. Aim for a minimum of three days a week of aerobic exercise, with no more than two days off between sessions.

Keep in mind that what we're trying to do is make sure that the heart is working hard enough. You're going to get all the aerobic benefits from that increase in heart rate, but also keep in mind that certain medications are going to make this not an accurate assessment. For example, if you take a beta blocker for heart disease, the bottom line is you're not going to fall into that zone, so you're going to have to ask your physician or cardiologist for a modification for you as an individual. So we've got aerobic. What about anaerobic?

"Anaerobic" means without oxygen. This is short lasting, high-intensity exercise, and this includes very heavy weight lifting, sprinting. You can always tell sprinters because again, they're going to cover a lot of distance in a very short period of time, so they may run that 100 in a very short period of time. That is an anaerobic event. Jumping rope, interval training, and isometrics are other examples. What are the benefits of these anaerobic exercises? It's the development of stronger muscles, and oftentimes, bigger muscles. So one of the things that happens in my practice is I deal with a lot of female sprinters. Because they sprint, because they're exercising without oxygen, they're an anaerobic athlete, the body adapts by making more muscle mass.

My sprinters will look and say, how did I end up with such large legs and a large behind? The body is adapting to the demand that you've placed on it. So it's a great example of the overload principle. You're asking the muscles to do more, i.e. sprint, and the only way it can do that is to adapt by increasing the muscle mass. Again, it makes you leaner and stronger, which adds in weight management, since muscles use more calories than fat.

For beginners who are not very fit, try interval training as a way to incorporate anaerobic exercise. For example, increase your running pace for a short period of time, so you might be running on the treadmill, and you're kind of jogging at maybe five miles per hour. Then for 10 to 60 seconds, you ramp up the speed, and then you bring it back down and have a slower recovery period. So that might be a way of you increasing your ability to tolerate sprinting activities.

Also part of this exercise plan must be flexibility. "Flexibility" means stretching muscle groups, and it increases range of motion and joints and muscles. It helps to protect our muscles and tissues from injuries or tears. Stretching after exercise can help keep the muscles in their maximum range of motion. Now, you notice that I said "after exercise." Stretching is not a warm-up. You do not take a cold muscle to its maximum stretching point. You want to be warmed up, so stretching should not be used as a warm-up. Now, say for example, you're going to go out and jog a little bit, maybe run around the parking lot one or two times, get your heart rate up, start to break a sweat, and then if you want to stretch before you go on your long run, it's perfectly okay. But stretching is not a warm-up.

What about hydration as part of this whole exercise plan? Dehydration can impair exercise performance and it can become life-threatening. Water deficits in excess of 2% to 3% of body weight can decrease exercise performance. Remember from our hydration lecture, for each pound you lose in physical activity, you've lost 16 ounces of sweat that you did not replace. In order to regain the fluid that you lost, you're going to need to replenish it with up to 16 to 24 ounces of extra fluid. So one of the challenges is I need you to weigh. Weighing before and after exercise is not going to assess how much body fat you lost. Keep in mind that in order to lose a pound of body fat, you have to lose 3500 calories. Chances are, in your exercise, you didn't run 35 miles, so the bottom line is that when you lose weight during exercise, it is always fluid weight.

Nutrition components. What should you eat before exercise? Well, low- to moderate-intensity exercise does not require extra food, and the problem that I see is people think, okay, I'm exercising. I need to eat more. What they actually do is they out-eat their exercise. So they might have walked three miles, burned about 300 calories, and then went out and ate a Big Mac, 600 calories, and lo and behold, they out-ate their exercise. But if you need something before exercise, a meal or a snack should provide you enough fluid to stay hydrated.

It should also be low in fat and fiber to minimize stomach problems. Yes, I did say "low in fiber," and dieticians do say things like "low in fiber." So your gut may not be able to tolerate extra fiber if you're going to go run or work out intensively. It should be, again, particularly if you're training aerobically, relatively high in carbohydrates to maintain blood sugar levels. It should be moderate in protein, but the key point is it has to be well tolerated by you. We're all a little bit different, so what might work for me might be a disaster for you.

What about during exercise? Well, during exercise, what you're really trying to do is replace the fluid losses and provide enough carbohydrate, particularly if you're doing an endurance workout. Think about if you're doing exercise for more than an hour, you're kind of running low on the carbohydrate tank, and you may need to have a source of carbohydrate. This would be a great time to have a sports drink. Also, you might want to consider levels of hydration and a need for calories in extremes of temperature, high heat or very low or high altitude.

What about after exercise? The most important thing is taking adequate fluids and energy, anything that's going to have calories and carbohydrate, to replace your storage carbohydrate, the carbohydrate that you had in the bank called your "muscle glycogen stores." So I think the challenge is a lot of it depends on how much time you're spending exercising. So again, if I go walk around my neighborhood, I do not need to eat before I exercise. I might want to have water during exercise, and I don't need to add more food after. So again, I think the key thing is the intensity of the exercise. Remember that FITT principle.

If I'm exercising intently, I really want to try and consume a small meal within about 30 minutes of physical activity to promote what's called "nutritional recovery." So what are some suggestions for food intake when you're on an exercise program? Well, this is, again, separate from the exercise experience. This is just part of your training diet. Increase the intake of whole grains, cereals, and legumes. Get five or more servings of fruits and vegetables a day. Keep in mind that these fruits and vegetables provide vitamins, minerals, fiber, and depending on the type of fruit or vegetable, they are between 80% and 90% water. So I describe it as the water that you chew. Consume adequate amounts of water throughout the day.

To personalize that exercise plan, it's important to develop a plan that feels right and will last for you. Change up different activities if you get bored throughout the week, and that might be a strategy. For me personally, I love doing the same thing all the time because as I push myself a little bit harder, I can monitor change over time. I can monitor my progress by doing something that's similar. Try resistance training every other day and do aerobic or anaerobic activities on the other days.

Maybe what you want to do is establish a walking or a running group with neighbors or coworkers. I usually recommend if you're going to do that, try and pick people that are about the same level of fitness you are. So if you're just a beginner, you don't want to go out and do a walking program with someone who competes in walking races. Also remember that what we're trying to do is make this enjoyable, so try gardening, dancing, biking, taking the stairs at work, if that's something that you can do.

There are a couple of ways to increase motivation to adhere to an exercise program. Get a pedometer. A pedometer can be used to track steps that you take every day and strive for at least 10,000 per day. But if you've not done this, don't start at 10,000. Maybe start a little bit lower, at about 2000 steps per day and work your way up. Do pedometers work? Research has been done to show how effective pedometers are. The results are improved motivation and readiness to exercise, and confidence for exercising. They will say that as you count your steps, you may oftentimes look at ways of adding more steps to your day. Certainly, there are pedometers out there that actually can help you to count your calories as well. Again, reductions in body weight, percent body fat, and waist circumference have also been shown with pedometer use. Get a partner to exercise with you if you need to be held accountable.

Keep in mind that you want to pick an activity that you like, not an activity that maybe your spouse likes. If you don't like that, the chances are you're not going to keep it up. So again, I think the key thing is whatever you do, pick out something that you like, and be consistent. Your body needs regular exposure to physical exercise. Exercise is medicine. You wouldn't stop taking your medicine, take a couple of days off and go back on it. I want you to think of exercise as medicine and get your daily dose.

What about some frequently asked questions? Do I have to do my half hour or hour of exercise all at one time? The science says no, you don't. Can I split it up? Absolutely, if it makes it more convenient. Say, for example, you've only got maybe 10 minutes to devote at lunch, then 10 minutes is part of that 30 that you might need to get for the day, and so maybe that 10 minute at lunch can help to make your exercise plan more sustainable.

Another frequently asked question is, should I exercise when I'm sick? The answer is no. You really need to take time off because if you're spending extra calories in energy for exercise, keep in mind that when you're ill, particularly when you have a fever, you have an increase in your metabolic rate and you body needs those calories for white blood cells, for the stress response. The bottom line is you need to take a couple of days off. Once you have an established exercise program, you know you're going to go back to it, but take some time off when you're sick. Also, be respectful. Don't go to a gym when you're ill because you've now exposed others in the gym as well.

Thank you very much.

The Future of Nutrition—Science and Trends
Lecture 35

What's on the horizon in the science of nutrition? ... Well, I don't have a crystal ball, but I do see some trends.

I want to begin with some exciting, cutting-edge scientific advances in nutrition. Nutritional genomics encompasses 2 fields: nutrigenetics and nutrigenomics. Nutrigenetics is a field in which nutritional interventions are planned around the genetic expression of a disease. Nutrigenomics is about eating for your genotype and includes the study of the impact of environmental factors on gene expression.

What is the significance of nutritional genomics? Common dietary substances can act on the human genome to alter gene expression or structure. Under certain circumstances in some individuals, diet can be a serious risk factor for a number of diseases. Some diet-regulated genes are likely to play a role in the onset, incidence, progression, and/or severity of some chronic illnesses.

The degree to which diet influences the balance between healthy and disease states may depend on the individual's genetic makeup. Dietary intervention based on the knowledge of a nutrition requirement, nutritional status, and genotype can be used to prevent, mitigate, or possibly cure chronic diseases.

Chronic diseases have become the leading concern of public health. Most of the common disorders are diet related. All of these disorders represent an imbalance. A specific and individualized approach to the treatment of these diseases is needed, and a solution may be in the near future.

Let's explore examples of gene-nutrient interaction discoveries. The *APOA1* gene codes for the main protein in HDL cholesterol; this data would give you information on the type of HDL variant that you possess and what would be the most beneficial intervention. The *LIPC* gene codes for the enzyme hepatic lipase. This determines your liver's ability to metabolize fat, which may determine if you will end up with fatty infiltration of the liver. In a study, women who consumed caffeine and had a variant of the vitamin D receptor (tt genotype) had considerably higher rates of bone loss than those who had the TT genotype.

Individuals with the *GSTT1*-null genotype who consume high levels of green tea do not have a protective effect against many forms of cancer.

What is the future of nutrigenomics? In reaction to findings, the functional food and nutrition supplement business will grow. More research is needed on the influence of specific nutrients on metabolic pathways and risk for chronic disease. This new approach of nutrient-gene interactions may redefine the practice of preventive medicine.

About 70% of American adults are attempting to consume healthier diets.

Another exciting new advance in the science of nutrition is metabolomics, which is a comprehensive profiling of individual metabolites, including food metabolites or metabolites in your own body processes. In the future, comprehensive direct assessment of your health will replace what we do now: looking at a single biomarker to treat disease.

Because metabolite information can change throughout a person's life, agreeing to have one's health evaluated through metabolomics may be an intermediary step between current practice and the use of nutrigenomics for assessing diet-related health concerns.

Metabolic changes in individuals are often due to environmental and lifestyle changes and aging. Possible health outcomes and vulnerabilities of individuals to metabolic stress may be predicted.

Let's look at some food-related trends. According to the Mintel Trends Study, about 70% of American adults are attempting to consume healthier diets. There are diverging trends: American consumers want something quick and easy, but we also want foods that go back to basics. The Mintel study shows us that we want homemade meals, so we need to integrate homemade and convenience. Using whole foods instead of highly processed foods is a popular trend. Choosing whole grains has also become a priority. Dairy, pork, and beef intake have been reduced, while fruit and vegetable consumption has increased.

Let's review some frequently asked questions. When do you think nutritional genomics and metabolomics will be viable options? We already have some of these advanced diagnostics available, and reliable testing may become more commonplace within 5 years.

Do you feel that metabolomics will be used to counter the effects of aging? Possibly, but the environment is always going to play a significant role.

New foods show up on the market shelves all the time. How can I tell if they are good for me and my family? Go back to the basics: Is it a whole food? Is it minimally processed?

Are we doing better or worse now than when you started your practice when it comes to our eating habits? I believe we are doing worse. ■

Suggested Reading

Brown, J., *Nutrition Now*, unit 34.

Kaput and Rodriguez, "Nutritional Genomics."

Questions to Consider

1. If nutritional genomics and metabolomics were standard approaches in health care today, what questions would you like answered?

2. Which food trend do you most appreciate: back to basics or convenience? Why?

The Future of Nutrition—Science and Trends
Lecture 35—Transcript

Greetings and welcome back. In my practice, I'm sometimes asked, "What's next? What's on the horizon in the science of nutrition?" The same topic often arises at professional conferences. Well, I don't have a crystal ball, but I do see some trends. So in this lecture, we're going to be discussing the future of nutrition. We'll talk a little bit more about consumer trends a bit later, but I want to tell you about some exciting, cutting-edge scientific advances in nutrition.

You've heard of the Human Genome Project, completed a number of years ago. This was an effort that identified all the 20,000 to 25,000 genes in the human DNA. Thanks to this project, the information that is available is beginning to integrate science and technology into the health-care arena for our population. That brings us to a word that maybe you haven't heard before, called "nutritional genomics," encompassing two fields, nutrigenetics and nutrigenomics. What are these terms? Let's define them.

"Nutrigenetics" is a field where the nutritional interventions are planned around the genetic expression of a disease. So you already know you have someone who has a genetically linked disease, and an example would be a disease called "phenylketonuria." This is a genetically transmitted disease, in which a specific dietary intervention, such as the manufacturing of a phenylalanine-free infant formula is the treatment. So we know what the disease is, and the treatment is designed around it.

"Nutrigenomics," simply stated, is eating for your genotype. It is the relationship between nutrition and specific nutrients with the functioning of the human genome. Think about it this way—your genes can determine whether eating a low-cholesterol or low-sodium diet for you as an individual will give the desired results. Your own genetic blueprint will truly give you a one-in-a-million diet prescription. So I want you to just think about the implications of that for a minute.

It also includes the study of the impact of environmental factors on gene expression. This could include age, diet, smoking, alcohol, and even things like region of the country. Think about vitamin D. You make more vitamin D in sunny climates than you do in cold climates. The convergence of these two terms and the information they provide are necessary to completely cover the benefits of nutritional genomics.

What is the significance? Common dietary substances can act on the human genome, either directly or indirectly, to alter gene expression or structure. Under certain circumstances in some individuals, diet can be a serious risk factor for a number of diseases. Think of this as your genetic crystal ball. As an example, if you have a genetic complement that increases your risk of type 2 diabetes, staying lean, avoiding becoming overly fat, and getting regular physical activity from childhood might be your prescription. You know what's in the future, and now you have the ability to modify it.

Some diet-regulated genes and their normal common variants are likely to play a role in the onset, incident, progression and/or severity of some chronic illnesses. So we might ask the question, who's most likely to develop cirrhosis of the liver? Not all individuals who consume the same amount of alcohol have the same progression. Similarly, not all individuals who become obese develop fatty infiltration of the liver. The secret code and the answer lie in your genes.

The degree to which diet influences the balance between healthy and disease states may depend on the individual's genetic makeup. Dietary intervention based on the knowledge of a nutrition requirement, a nutritional status, and your genotype—remember that individualized nutrition—can be used to prevent, mitigate, or even possibly cure chronic diseases. Throughout this series, you haven't heard me say "cure disease," but this might be the avenue by which we're able to do that. This will add a new and personal component to the nutrition assessment process. In our lecture on creating your own nutrition plan, we talked about the ABC and D of assessment, and now genes can add the "G" to that alphabet.

Those chronic diseases just mentioned have become the leading health concerns of public health. Most of the common disorders are diet related, and certainly, examples would include cancers, cardiovascular disease, diabetes, neurological disorders, obesity, osteoporosis, and other inflammatory disorders. All of these disorders represent an imbalance in homeostasis, which just means the balance of the normal functioning of the body. They are linked to not only environmental but diet factors as the cause.

Some of us are far more sensitive to environmental changes and may increase the inflammatory response linked with many diseases. A specific and individualized approach to the treatment of these diseases is needed, and a solution may be in the near future. So again, you wouldn't go to a dietician and get the same 1200-calorie diet that he or she may prescribe for somebody else. You would get a customized program. Genetic outcomes, however, are usually modified through the interaction of genetic variations and environmental factors. So please keep in mind the environment is always going to play a role in genetic expression.

For example, you may have a budding marathon runner in your family, who really doesn't like running long distances. The training he enjoys may ultimately determine his genetic outcome, so again, we've got to marry environment and genetic expression. Examples of some of the gene-nutrient interaction discoveries include cholesterol. We've talked a lot about cholesterol throughout this course. A gene has been identified called "APOA1" that codes for the main protein in HDL cholesterol. This gene has a vital role in lipid metabolism. If you have this data at your hand, this data would give you information on the type of HDL variant that you possess and that predominates in your blood, and what would be the most beneficial, if any, intervention.

Traditionally now, for individuals who have low HDL, we prescribe the same thing. This would change the prescription of the modification of that HDL variant. We have also talked about lipids as well. The LIPC gene, an enzyme that binds and uptakes lipoproteins, codes for the enzyme hepatic lipase. This determines your liver's ability to metabolize fat. Again, that may determine who's going to end up with fatty infiltration of the liver.

Let's look at a few more. Caffeine was studied as a risk factor for bone loss in elderly women. In the results of this study, women who consume more than 300 milligrams of caffeine, about three cups or 24 ounces of coffee a day, and had a variant of the vitamin D receptor (tt genotype) had considerably higher rates of bone loss than those who had the TT genotype.

So I think again, your genetic variation is going to determine whether or not you're going to be the one that's vulnerable to bone loss. So this data for an individual would give servings and amounts of caffeine that might be tolerated before the onset of bone loss.

We have information about green tea and cancer. Observations have shown that individuals who consume high levels of green tea have a protective effect against many forms of cancer. We discussed this in our lecture on nutrition and cancer. However, this is not the case for individuals carrying the GSTT1-null genotype. These people lack a particular enzyme involved in detoxification, so people with this null genotype would be advised to use other food sources for any kind of detoxification process. So that's almost a strange new world, isn't it?

What is the future of nutrigenomics? It is predicted that in reaction to findings in nutritional genomics research, the functional food and nutrition supplement business will considerably grow in the next decade or so. More research is needed on the influence of specific nutrients on metabolic pathways and risk for chronic disease. Research focus, and I think this is a key point, might need to be refined to control for genetic variation. Right now, our closest association is looking at ethnic groups. I live in south Texas, where there is Starr County, which is unique in the fact that a good percentage of people who are born there don't ever leave. So they have a relatively homogenous genetic pool. It's one of the most common places in the United States to study, for example, diabetes, because the gene pool has remained intact in Starr County.

This new approach of nutrient-gene interactions may redefine the current practice of what we call "preventive medicine" today. So what are some key points that you could think about? Dieticians armed with all this data could specifically tailor their message to each individual, based on that individual's outcome of gene interactions and nutrient intake. This method would allow people in turn to tailor their dietary and lifestyle decisions.

The success is oftentimes going to depend on adequate communication among health-care providers and researchers, as well as the correct dissemination of information to the community and to consumers. So you can imagine how this information might be received. What's going to happen to the diet book industry, for example? If indeed we're all unique individuals, the sales of those books may be tailored, and you might see some new things appear on your bookshelves.

Another exciting new advance in the science of nutrition is metabolomics, again, another word that you're probably not familiar with. Defined by researchers by the name of German, Watkins, and Fay, metabolomics is a comprehensive profiling of individual metabolites, which can be food metabolites, or they can certainly be metabolites in your own body processes, which are linked to an understanding of health and human metabolism. As with nutritional genomics, the science is emerging to provide people with unique individualized health goals, based on their own metabolic profile.

This means that the prevention of metabolic illness is more than just steering people away from current health problems. It means our focus could change, and now we would direct metabolism in an individual way towards an optimal personal metabolic state. Dietary health is contingent on more than just genetics, so using genotype alone will not be enough to assess someone's personal health status.

What's our key point with this? In the future, comprehensive direct assessment of your health will replace what we do now, which is looking at a single biomarker to treat disease. For example, we currently look at your cholesterol for heart disease, and your glucose for diabetes. What we might look at in the future is to expand this a little bit larger and say, how do you as an individual respond to inflammation? How do you as an individual respond to other things in terms of glucose for the management of diabetes? So I always say, stay tuned for more developments.

Metabolite information, unlike genetic information, can change throughout a person's life, due to aging, diet, and other lifestyle choices. So what might be true in terms of your metabolic profile when you're 20 may not be true when you're 50. Because of this, agreeing to have one's health evaluated through metabolomics may be an intermediary step between current practice and the use of nutrigenomics for assessing diet-related health concerns. Well, what might the benefits of metabolomics be?

It will be a complete personalized, individual view of your metabolism revealed through this method. Think of those individuals who struggle to lose weight. This might be the answer to the question for that individual person. Is my weight solely inherited or is it mostly environmental? So think about this. You may have a genetic predisposition to becoming obese, but as you go through the life cycle, your metabolites and your blood change, and now the weight loss plan that worked for you in your 20s needs to be modified and customized for you as you age. Metabolic changes in individuals are oftentimes, again, due to environmental and lifestyle changes and aging. These can be identified by this new process.

Possible health outcomes and vulnerabilities of individuals to metabolic stress may be predicted. Now, with all of this, we have to stop and reflect about the ethics in this emerging science. So what are some of the things to consider? Although this sounds so wonderful, we have to step back and think, what might the consequence be? One of the things we have to consider is, how are we going to secure and safeguard confidentiality? What about ensuring privacy rights? What about facing the discrimination regarding insurance coverage and employment?

If an insurance provider understands that you are at significantly greater risk of heart disease or significantly greater risk of diabetes, will employment discrimination emerge? Other problems regard dealing with the genetic examination of children and some of the limits of parental authority, and deciding whether you as an individual want to share this personal information with other family members. So that's, again, the strange new world of what's coming in the future in terms of that diet and disease relationship.

I think we can change our focus and start to take a look at some food-related trends. What are consumers interested in in the future? Well, according to the Mintel Trends Study, which is a consumer survey, about 70% of U.S. adults are attempting to consume healthier diets. Most consumers are interested in nutrition, and try and make healthy choices when purchasing products. What about consumer preferences? As we have seen, science suggests that advanced diagnostics are on the way, but trends of American eating patterns still drive food selection and market-driven products. So again, the Mintel study shows us these trends.

What was learned seems to indicate diverging trends. We as American consumers want something that's quick and easy, but we also want this back to basics. We want, again, maybe a little bit more holistic approach to nutrition. What are some of the things in convenience that American consumers want? We want portability and we want one-handed consumption. Well, I'm always a little concerned about this one-handed consumption, so does that mean we want to have foods that we can drive with? Does this mean we want to be able to multitask at our desks and eat our lunch in one hand and type with another? But we certainly want things that are convenient.

It's also on the rise in many families with young children who are always on the go. I certainly remember when my son played high school soccer. I worked fulltime and we ate a lot of sandwich dinners at 10 o'clock at night because I didn't have everything convenient that I needed to have to fix a home-cooked dinner when we got home so late. We also want ways of bringing a restaurant experience into our home, and you might notice this when you go to the grocery store right now.

Some examples include things like microwaveable Panini sandwiches, some of the gourmet frozen pasta dinners for families, like chicken broccoli fettuccine alfredo. Things that you would normally get in a restaurant are now kind of emerging to the American table. Customer convenience in packaging and preparation—we now have resealable cookie and cracker packages, plastic, reusable lunch meat containers, microwaveable packages of frozen vegetables that are already pre-seasoned for us. We want convenience, but we also want this back to basics trend.

Many consumers have seemed to reverse their food consumption patterns. Even the Mintel study showed a focus on cooking homemade meals versus convenience products. I will tell you, in my family, my daughter always played sports growing up in high school, and so she goes to college and she calls me and says, "Mom, I really need to know how to heat up a LEAN CUISINE dinner." I said, "Well, you just pop it in the microwave." She said, "But is it microwaveable safe?" And it taught me that she not only didn't really know convenience foods, but she certainly didn't know how to make a home-cooked meal. So now we're seeing on television cooking channels and other things that are teaching us to make things that are almost homemade.

So I think the Mintel study is showing us that we want homemade meals, but we might want to integrate homemade and convenience.

Some consumers are not using all the new and improved products. They're going back to basics and purchasing whole foods and cooking at home. We've discussed in previous lectures the resurgence of the farmers' market in terms of bringing people some fresher produce to their table. Others, again, are participating in growing their own produce through home gardens or herb gardens, or being involved in community garden projects. The challenge, however, is to oftentimes marry the desire to have all of these more natural-type products with our hectic American lifestyle. So using whole foods instead of highly-processed foods is a trend that's becoming popular among all populations. The question is, how do we get that done?

When we think, okay, we want convenience and portability, but I also want homemade, doesn't this conflict? Aren't these conflicting messages? But actually, if you think about it, these trends actually converge. For example, I will admit I purchase precut vegetables to make a stir fry at home, so I like the convenience of precut fresh, but I also have to have something that's homemade. I like that homemade flavor. Try combining precut or frozen fruits and yogurt for making your own homemade smoothies. Again, one of my favorite things to do is take a bag of frozen fruit, semi-defrosted, put it in a food processor with a carton of yogurt, and now I've got a smoothie that will rival any of the companies that are out there. So we want convenience and we want freshness at the same time. If I'm a marketing agent, I'm going to look at getting these two trends to marry.

According to the *Nutrition and You: Food Trends* survey, choosing whole grains has also become a priority. Ninety-four percent of respondents in this survey stated whole grains are healthier than refined carbohydrates, so that whole grain message is out. So you'll see food manufacturers that are trying to come up with unique front-of-package labeling to manage that consumer trend. Additionally, respondents in the study said that they have reduced their intake of dairy, pork, and beef. It is unclear whether this is just wellness-driven to avoid saturated fat, or if it is economically driven. These are very high cost sources of protein, and again, it could be both or one. We don't really have all the data on that.

Consumers are reporting increasing consumption of fruits and vegetables. This shift in food choice will influence the directions of sustainability, nutrition counseling, as well as the health conditions of the population. So when we look at the future of nutrition, what we're really looking at is, what does the science say is up and coming? And what are we doing now? What are Americans interested in now? I think, again, that summarizes nicely the future of nutrition.

Onto those frequently asked questions. When do you think nutritional genomics and metabolomics will be viable options in the toolkits of health professionals? Again, this is really looking into the crystal ball. Clearly, the trend exists now in examining the outcome of genetic expression with advance lipid analysis. There's a company in the United States, and there are many, but this is just one called the "Berkeley Heart Health Labs," and it does just this. It subfractionates LDL and HDL into its individual types to learn a little bit more about the type of carrier protein, and oftentimes, the carrier protein, is it very effective at getting rid of the cholesterol or is the carrier protein ineffective, and now that LDL gets deposited into arterial walls?

We already have some of this advanced diagnostics available, and again, what it's looking at is the genetic expression of the protein subtypes that are going to be responsible for transporting LDL and HDL to their respective delivery points. We also can see genetic testing for athletic performance, and that's already available as well, suggesting that you can determine your muscle fiber type predisposition. This would supposedly tell parents if their offspring could run marathons or if they'd be better suited to running sprints. Certainly, there are countries in the world that already use some of this testing to decide who does what in the Olympics. So again, although you might think of this as a strange new world, there are things out there.

I'm also going to remind you about the ethical dilemmas associated with that. So I think the real challenge is if indeed you had a son or daughter who was genetically gifted to run sprints, but they hated that, forcing them into an event that they didn't like or enjoy would really take away some of the pleasure of sports. There are some companies offering those kinds of services now, but reliable interventions may be available on a more regular basis within the next five years. So again, stay tuned.

Another frequently asked question is do you feel that metabolomics will be used to counter the effects of aging? Well, possibly, but it also raises some questions. Say, for example, what you could do in your 20s. Your metabolites in your blood are saying, I can lose weight like this in my 20s, but I can't in my 50s. What if you can't lose weight, despite not being genetically behind the eight ball? I'm understanding this and thinking, okay, wait a minute. Metabolomics is saying I should be able to lose this weight, but I can't.

I think oftentimes what we're missing here is the environment is always going to play a significant role. Just because your metabolomics is saying, yeah, you can lose weight this way, the challenge is if you don't account for the environment, you may not be able to get the desired results. I think when we look at this, you always have to think, yes, this is going to give us more data, but it isn't necessarily going to solve all the problems if indeed we also don't look at that environmental expression.

As we look at food trends, another question that I get is, new foods show up on the market shelves all the time. How can I tell if they're good for me and my family? Well, I always suggest going back to the basics. Following that Mintel survey, go back to the basics. Is it a whole food? Is it minimally processed? Again, I think the challenge is trying to integrate convenience along with that. So again, the more hands that touch it, the more items on the ingredient list, the more likely it is to be not as healthy as a minimally processed food.

Another question. "You mentioned that food choices will influence the direction of health conditions of a population. In your view, are we doing better or worse than when you started your practice when it comes to our eating habits?" Actually, I believe we're doing worse. We're always saying, well, I don't understand why I'm overweight. When I first started in clinical practice, I didn't see the degree of obesity that I see now. The largest person in my practice that I've ever taken care of is over 1000 pounds, and when I started a long time ago, almost 30 years ago, I didn't see this. And I now consider obesity the tsunami of public health diseases because obesity is linked with heart disease and cancer. So actually, I think it's worse.

I think both our genetic expression and metabolomics will give us more answers to this dilemma. But again, I think in terms of a public health strategy, when we're talking about obesity, we really have to look at both global and individual strategies because I don't think we can look at just the genetic blueprint and say, "That's going to be the magic bullet of weight loss." We're also going to have to take a look at environmental issues as well.

Thank you very much.

Nutrition Facts and FAQs
Lecture 36

Nutrition is a very broad and very personal subject. After all, we make choices about our diet and our family's diet every day, several times a day.

For the most part, we have ended the past 35 lectures with frequently asked questions regarding the lecture topic. This last lecture is devoted to some of the common questions about nutrition that I have been asked during my years as a registered dietician and professor of nutrition.

Let's start with some general questions. What is a nutrition counselor or dietician? A nutritionist can be anyone interested in nutrition, but a registered dietician has completed at least a 4-year degree and an internship, so that is the kind of health-care provider you are looking for. How do you find a good registered dietician? Ask for recommendations from friends or try the American Dietetic Association's website.

What should you consider when consulting with a dietician? Look at whether you connect with them, and make sure they do a thorough nutrition assessment.

Upon diagnosis of a disorder or condition that is affected by diet, what should I look for? Look for someone who is a specialist in that area of nutrition.

What information do I need to bring along? Bring any pertinent information. Write down what you normally eat and the times of day that you struggle.

What do you like best about being a dietician? The thing that makes this career choice fresh and interesting is no 2 people are the same.

What changes have you seen in the science of nutrition since you first began your practice? At first, it was about foods. About midway, it was about vitamins and minerals. Now it is a bit retro, back to whole foods.

Let's look at some diet and nutrition questions. What are the risks and benefits of being vegetarian? It is great to get more vegetables; the challenge is knowing enough about protein sources.

I became vegetarian to lose weight, so why have I gained weight? Keep in mind that calories rule and are always going to count—certain foods, like cheese and nuts, are high in calories.

Everybody in my family wants a different diet, so what is the best approach to meet their goals? Your core meals can be the same, but you can dress them up differently.

I got almost a million hits in an Internet search for herbs and weight loss. Are there any that work? Yes, but their safety is questionable.

Let's look at some nutrition and lifestyle questions. How do I break the unhealthy habit of eating a lot toward the end of the day? Recognize that the science says people do better eating 3 meals and maybe a snack in between; recognize where you are most vulnerable.

What do you think about black cohosh for the treatment of menopause symptoms? There is some evidence that it may be effective for hot flashes, but the purity and safety of supplements like these are not regulated, so it is a personal decision.

Can nutrition drinks make up for protein my aging mother does not eat? They can be useful, but taste fatigue may occur if she drinks them regularly. Always look for a whole food approach.

Are protein powders to build muscles beneficial or harmful? They can be beneficial. Just remember you still have to do the strength training to build muscle.

Is whey protein worth the cost? Whey protein is milk protein, so you can get it cheaper and more conveniently in milk.

Does the military provide a well-balanced diet in their meals that are ready to eat (MREs)? Yes, a great team of dieticians helped to design the MREs based on various activity levels.

Do you have any suggestions for someone who is worried that if she quits smoking, she will gain a lot of weight? Part of the addiction to smoking is the oral fixation. Try replacing it with air-popped popcorn or chewing gum.

Let's look at some beverage and nutrition questions. What are the long-term impacts of diet soda and its associated chemicals on our health? Nonnutritive sweeteners have been determined to be safe, but for long-term safety, always stick to moderation.

Are vitamin waters good for you? Very few people actually have vitamin deficiencies, and the majority of vitamin waters and flavor-enhanced waters contain some form of sugar—is this something you really want to drink?

Let's look at some disorder and nutrition questions. Is there such a thing as too little stomach acid? Yes, it is called achlorhydria. People think of stomach acid as a bad thing, but we need it.

My parents have lost their sense of taste as they have aged. Is there anything that I can do to improve their eating? Make sure that their food is flavorful.

Here are some final tips.

- Eat for balance and color.

- Watch out for shiny foods.

- Watch your portion size.

- Eat like a child.

- Move.

- Good nutrition is essential nutrients in the right amount plus the foods you love because you are you. ∎

Questions to Consider

1. What question would you have for Professor Anding?

2. Which health-care professional would be best able to answer your question—a physician, a dietician, a pharmacist, a personal trainer, or someone else?

Nutrition Facts and FAQs
Lecture 36—Transcript

Hello, and welcome back to the last lecture in this series. For the most part, we have ended the past 35 lectures with a short FAQ, or frequently asked questions, session to answer the questions I'm often asked about regarding the lecture topic. Nutrition is a very broad and very personal subject. After all, we make choices about our diet and our family's diet every day, several times a day. Many nutrition questions can remain. That's why we'll be devoting this last lecture to responding to some of the common questions about nutrition that I have been asked during my years as a registered dietician and a Professor of Nutrition.

Let's start with some general questions that I believe many of you might have had. What does a nutrition counselor or a dietician do? I'm first going to start out by correcting the nomenclature. You are a "nutritionist" because you're interested in nutrition. That's the definition. There is a difference between the definition of a "nutritionist" and a "registered dietician." A registered dietician must go to college, complete a four-year degree and at minimum, do an internship, where he or she can apply what they've learned in the classroom to the real world. So when you're going out and looking and someone's saying, "I'm a nutritionist" you also want to ask them, "are you also a registered dietician?" So a registered dietician is the right kind of health-care provider that you would look for.

How do you find a good one? Just like you'd find a good doctor. Sometimes you can ask a friend, "Oh, by the way, have you been to a dietician?" "Yeah, I had a really great one. He or she helped me to lose weight." If that's not within your friend's purview, they had not ever seen a registered dietician, you can go to the website of the American Dietetic Association, which is www.eatright.org, and you can find a dietician in your area. But I want you to keep in mind here that just as physicians have become specialized—you have obstetricians, you have pediatricians, you have internists—dieticians are also specialized. If you're really looking for a pediatric dietician, that's the kind of person that you want to request. So when you're looking through that list of registered dieticians, look at someone who might practice in a large pediatric hospital. So again, you're looking for a registered dietician, not a nutritionist, and look for a subspecialist in the area that you're interested in.

What should an individual consider when they're consulting with a dietician? Well, I'm going to suggest to you that you want to take a look at whether or not you can connect with this person. Because nutrition is really very personal, you want someone who's going to understand you, your family lifestyle, things that you do, things that you're interested in doing, so you want to make sure that you have someone that you connect with. You can also expect to spend about an hour, maybe an hour and a half, with someone, who's going to, first and foremost, do a nutrition assessment to see where you're starting. They will help you formulate goals, negotiate goals with you, and come up with an action plan when you walk out the door.

I usually will describe to my clients my first visit with them is, we're going to get started, but it may take me more than one visit to understand your barriers, what's making this plan work for you, and why it's great, or where maybe I missed something on the assessment, or I didn't ask a right question, and now we have to modify that goal.

Another question is upon a diagnosis of a disorder or a condition that's affected by diet, now what should I look for? What you're looking for is someone who's a specialist in that area. I will tell you, it's been a long time since I've worked in an intensive care unit, so I wouldn't be the person to give you advice on a truly critical illness. Because my practice is on weight management, and pediatrics, and sports, I might be the kind of person that you would want to employ during that period of time.

Another frequently asked question is, if I'm going to invest my valuable time and my valuable resources seeing a dietician, what information do I need to bring along? This, actually, is a really brilliant question because you want to maximize that time with that person. You don't want to have them say, "Well, what's your cholesterol?" "I don't know. I've got that at home. I didn't think about it." Bring any pertinent information. If you've had a BOD POD done, for example, to assess your body fat, bring that along with you.

An invaluable take-along is to write down what you normally eat. Remember, this is all about making progress, not perfection. Write down what you normally eat and areas of the day that you might struggle. Write down a three-day diet history before you go. Keep in mind that sometimes we eat a little differently Monday through Friday. Saturday and Sunday, we do something different. So I want you to think about, how does my weekend vary from my weekday? And maybe you give me one day that's a weekend, and two days that are weekdays. So keep in mind what you're trying to do is make this experience with a registered dietician as personal as you can.

I'm also going to take this opportunity to answer a question that I've never been asked before, but that I would really like to answer. What do you like best about being a dietician? Well, honestly, the science of nutrition is intriguing and fascinating to me, but what I like the best are people. So everybody's going to bring a little bit different spin, so the thing that makes this, as a career choice, fresh and interesting is no two people are the same. They're not going to have the same barriers, the same preferences, and so that makes my job unbelievably exciting and something that I look forward to doing every single day.

Another great question: Are there certain websites for women or men that you would recommend? Again, a lot of it depends on what your individual goal is. So if you said to me, "You know, I would really like to become fitter," then I would say to you, "Go to the American College of Sports Medicine website, www.ACSM.org, and again, learn how to find a professional in your area." If you're looking for something like a fun nutrition tip of the day, you can certainly go to www.eatright.org and have a nutrition tip sent to your computer on a daily basis.

If you're looking for more specific information, if you're looking for something that's more disease tailored, keep in mind that if you put in a Google search, or an Internet search, for diabetes, you're going to come up with a lot of things that are great, but a lot of things that are not so great. So how do you refine that? Well, go to governmental sites. So for example, you may want to go to the National Institutes of Health if you're looking for really great and reliable information on diabetes. If you're looking for reliable and great information on cancer, go to the websites of the big cancer centers in the United States. It could be Sloan-Kettering. In my area of the world, it's MD Anderson. So you can go to those websites and again, get really great information tailored for that disease.

Another frequently asked question is what changes have I seen in the science of nutrition since I first began my practice? When I first began, we really talked mostly about food, and not so much about the individual nutrients. Kind of midway through my practice, we all jumped on the, "It's the vitamin and mineral" bandwagon, and you started to see dieticians, including myself, recommend that everybody take vitamin E, or that vitamin C was going to be the great solution for the common cold. And as a lot of the research has been refined and explored in a little bit more depth, what I'm now seeing is almost that retro idea of going back to whole food.

In this series, we've talked about wonderful things, wonderful compounds in fruits and vegetables with names that we can't pronounce. It's not just the pigments in fruits and vegetables. It is truly the whole food that makes us well. It's not an individual nutrient. So basically, we are getting back to basics. Mother Nature knew best, and all the things that we need to be healthy and well actually belong in the whole food, not the processed food, but the whole food.

Under the category of nutrition and diets, and again, diet is one of these things that always is on everybody's mind, and I'm going to first and foremost refine that word for you. A "diet" is what you eat. You can modify that diet to meet a particular interest of yours or a health goal of yours, but diet doesn't necessarily imply weight reduction. So as we look at frequently asked questions, what are the risks and benefits of being vegetarian? Is it a healthy lifestyle? Can I get sufficient protein and other nutrients?

There are some real benefits associated with being vegetarian. Almost by definition, you're going to be getting more vegetables, maybe alternative sources of protein, like beans and nuts, so you are going to be gravitating towards what we know to be healthy, a plant-based diet. The challenge is, do you know enough about protein and its food sources? Can you get enough? And again, vegetarians have a wide variety of tools in their toolbox. Beans and rice would be a great source of protein for a vegetarian. A peanut butter and jelly sandwich on wholegrain bread is another great source of protein. You could do tofu in a rice dish, giving you another great source of protein.

It's when you really refine that further and become a vegan that you get yourself into a little bit of a dilemma. Getting sufficient protein on a vegetarian diet is not a problem, but remember, when I create a nutrient hole, I must address it. If I don't have any animal protein in my diet, animal protein houses vitamin B_{12}. So you can certainly be vegetarian, but if you drink milk and eat yogurt, there's your B_{12}. If you're vegetarian and you really have no animal protein in your diet, you're also going to be missing vitamin B_{12}, so keep that in mind.

One of my favorite questions is, "You know what, I became vegetarian to lose weight, but I've gained." Keep in mind that calories rule, and so if your goal is to become vegetarian, and you're not eating traditional meat any more, but you've now added all the cheese in the world, cheese is going to be 100 calories an ounce. Lo and behold, I see a lot of people becoming vegetarian that lost sight of the concept that yes, vegetarianism is a very healthy plan, absolutely a healthy plan. The challenge is, I still have to worry about calories, and so calories are always going to count on any kind of plan.

If you think, well, I'm not eating cheese, are you eating hummus? This is chickpeas and oftentimes oil is added to it. Are you eating nuts? One of my favorite things to tell people is that a cup of nuts has about 600 calories. Think of how easy it would be to grab a handful of nuts here and there, and all of a sudden, you've got more calories than you would have gotten if you'd eaten meat. Health benefits are different, but I think the challenge is if you're vegetarian and you want to lose weight, you also have to control sources of fat in your diet.

Another frequently asked question is, everybody in my family wants a different diet. My daughter's trying to lose weight. My son's trying to gain for wrestling. My husband wants gourmet meals, and I need to cook quickly. Now, the hard part here is no one, and I truly mean no one, can be a short-order cook for everyone in their family, and quite honestly, I don't think that's the best approach. You would think of it this way. Say, for example, you've got all kinds of different goals in your family, some people trying to gain, some people trying to lose. Your core meals can be the same.

For example, everybody, whether they're trying to gain or lose, should try to have 50% of their plate fruits and vegetables. If your husband wants a gourmet meal, 50% of that plate still needs to be fruits and vegetables. The way that you dress it up and the way that you don't end up being a short-order cook is maybe on the other side, say for example, it's a pasta dish. For you, you may want pasta with marinara. You don't want all the oil. Your daughter wants pasta with marinara because she's trying to lose weight, but lo and behold, your son needs some additional calorie support. This is where you can fortify that food with olive oil. Just take out yours, add a little bit of olive oil, put some on your son's plate, and everybody's essentially eating the same thing. Now, your husband may not be so happy, and maybe you all can take a cooking class together to make sure that he can learn how to cook as well as you.

Another asked question, I did an Internet search for herbs and weight loss, and got almost a million hits. Well, keep in mind that Americans are weight loss and diet focused, so it shouldn't surprise you that this is going to give you a lot of hits. Are there any that work? The short answer to that is yes, there are ones that work, but are they safe? That's where we have to put the big question mark. Certainly, there have been studies done, looking at the combination of ephedra and caffeine as a weight loss strategy, two herbal products, two plant-based products. It is effective, no doubt about it. However, if you have high blood pressure, or if you can't trust the purity and the safety of the herb that you got, you're not necessarily getting it from a big company—the value of that is yes, you might be able to lose weight, but at what cost?

I always look at this as a teaching moment. If you are really interested in losing weight and you're looking for an alternative way to do it, maybe that alternative way for you needs to be a little bit more exercise and some smaller portions. I know you've heard that before, but not being able to peek into your body, I get really concerned with the lack of purity and safety in the dietary supplement industry to say I could guarantee with 100% effectiveness that you wouldn't have an adverse reaction. And so my recommendation is although there may be some science to support the herbs, we have to stop short at brands and say which ones are safe. And to be honest with you, I don't know that I can safely answer that question for you.

As we get into the nutrition and lifestyle category, oftentimes, what you hear is, "You know what, I'm so busy in the morning or I don't have an appetite. I do kind of eat a reasonable lunch and maybe a healthy snack, but I work late and I arrive home and I'm ravenous. I eat a great deal just before I go to bed. I've heard this is called "crescendo eating," highlights at the end of the day, on television. Other than quitting my job, how can I break this unhealthy habit?" Well, I'm pretty fond of saying that when I get that hungry, I would eat anything, and this is what I do for a living. So you have to realize if you allow yourself to get that hungry, if you don't balance your food intake, breakfast, lunch, dinner, and maybe a snack in between, if you don't do that, biology rules.

This is not a question of willpower, and almost every time you see a diet commercial on television, it says, "You need to have more willpower." But if you're skipping meals or you're eating a little bit during the day and you get home in the afternoon, most of us are going to over-consume. So I look at this as biology, not willpower. So if that is you, first and foremost, we know individuals who eat breakfast every day generally weigh less than their breakfast-skipping counterparts. So on your action plan, it might be, can I get you something small at breakfast? Then after you've completed your own little nutrition assessment, you recognize your most vulnerable period is about that 30 minutes before you walk in the door.

I'll tell you how I handle this. Just like you, I work long hours. I spend a lot of time at work, and if I am running late and I'm not going to get home till eight o'clock at night, I pop popcorn and eat it in my car on the way home. If not, I'm going to walk in the door so hungry that I will pick a whole dinner before I actually sit down and eat my dinner. So I think the challenge is to recognize that the science says people do better with breakfast, lunch, dinner, and maybe a snack in between, and to recognize where you, as an individual, are most vulnerable. If that's right when you walk in the door, maybe your snack in the afternoon needs to be in your car right on the way home.

Nutrition choices and challenges.: Again, a frequently asked question, "My sister-in-law swears by black cohosh for the treatment of hot flashes and other signs of menopause, but I'm doubtful. What do you think?" Again, there's a disconnect here between the science. There is some science to suggest that black cohosh may be effective for hot flashes. The question is, "Can you get a reliable brand?" So again, the disconnect that we have here in the United States is the purity and the safety of the brand. As an individual, if you're willing to risk the fact that maybe you don't have as much active ingredient in your dietary supplement, but you feel so much better that you're willing to take the risk and take black cohosh, then I would say that really looks like one of those things that falls into that personal decision. There's not necessarily a right or a wrong. It becomes a personal decision. What is most important to you?

Another frequently asked question is, "My aging mother eats very little protein. Meat is difficult for her to chew, and she just doesn't enjoy it as much as she used to. Isn't it harmful? What about nutrition drinks like Ensure to make up for what she doesn't eat?" Keep in mind that we always want to look for a whole food approach. Although Ensure and a lot of the other nutrition drinks are nutritious by definition, what can happen, particularly in the elderly, is you can end up with what's called "taste fatigue." Now, I will say, I love oatmeal, but if I had to eat oatmeal 365 days of the year for breakfast and that's all I had, at some point in time, the oatmeal's not delicious. And so Ensure can fall into that same kind of trap. It's not that she might not like it in the beginning, but the problem is can she do it every day?

What you're looking at is the barrier that she might have to consumption of protein-containing foods is maybe she can't chew it. Are there softer protein alternatives? How about this? What about scrambled eggs? Add a little bit of cheese to it. Make it taste like something that's unbelievably nutritious and delicious, and something that is a whole food. Keep in mind that even the yellow in the yolk, although the yolk contains most of the cholesterol, contains lutein, and so there's some additional nutrition in that egg, as well as the protein, that Ensure may not be able to provide. So again, it's not harmful to use these nutrition drinks, but always look for a whole food alternative.

Another alternative for someone who just doesn't like the taste of meat or think it tastes odd: This is, again, a time to partner up with your pharmacist. Is she having changes in her taste secondary to a medication that she's taking? Is there an alternative choice? Is she having changes in her taste because she actually has a nutrient deficiency? Zinc, for example, will cause an alteration in taste and may be the reason the food doesn't taste delicious any more has nothing to do with the food itself, but a nutrient hole that your mother has.

Because I deal with athletes, this is a very popular question in my world. "My teenage son and his friends drink protein powders to build muscle. Are those products beneficial, harmful, worth the cost?" First and foremost, a couple of key points here. Puberty doesn't happen to everybody at the exact same time, so the bottom line is a 15-year-old male is not a 15-year-old male. There are going to be some 15-year-old men, and I mean men, who look like men, and then there are 15-year-old boys who really look like boys. So the challenge is the individuals who are more likely to use protein powders and dietary supplements to build muscle are not who you think. In my practice, it's the individuals who are trying to look like the 15-year-old men, but are still 15-year-old boys.

Protein powders by themselves do not build muscle. You have to create an anabolic stimulus, so for young men or young women or any of us who are trying to build muscle, protein doesn't build muscle unless the anabolic stimulus—weight training, strength training—is present. So are they beneficial? Sure they can be beneficial. They're a convenient source of protein. You can oftentimes take these protein powders or products with you to the gym and feed the muscles right after you're done exercising to help to build new mass. But the problem is the harm comes when an individual believes that this is going to be muscles in a bottle. It doesn't work that way. You really have to have a whole complete package.

When someone says, my son wants to buy whey protein. Is it worth the cost? I'll remind you again about your nursery rhymes. Little Miss Muffet sat on her tuffet, eating her curds and whey. Whey protein is milk protein. The curd in milk is casein, so most of the muscle-building products on the market are whey protein and you can get it in milk. So a great recovery drink for your son or daughter who's lifting weights is actually chocolate milk. Chocolate for the sugar, which helps to stimulate insulin production, and if you remember, insulin takes food out of the blood into the muscle where it can be used. So you want a little sugar after you're done lifting. And chocolate milk, how delicious is that? Again, it's in every high school cafeteria, so it'd be something that would be a way to minimize the cost and still get the benefits.

Another question is, my son is in the service overseas under rigorous conditions. Is he really getting a well balanced diet eating the meals that are ready to eat, the MREs? Is there something that we can send to him to supplement his diet that's not going to spoil in the mail? The great news about our military is they actually have a great team of dieticians behind the scenes who help to design the MREs, based on the level of activity that your son might get. So there is a lot of science going into those MREs. Again, this is an example where you have to modify the food to fit the environment. The problem is you have to keep the food safe to eat, so oftentimes, fresh foods are off the table because they're going to spoil.

That means you, as a parent, might struggle to send him something to supplement his diet that isn't going to spoil in the mail. For my military friends, they'll tell me they love getting things like power bars and energy bars in the mail because, again, that might be something that adds a little flavor variety. Depending on how you ship it, you can actually send nuts and dried fruit, and again, that dried fruit is going to have a lot of the really beneficial phytonutrients in it. It's just in a more shelf-stable form.

Another question: "My sister is a heavy smoker, but she is worried that if she quits smoking, she will gain a lot of weight. Have you got any suggestions for her from a nutritional standpoint?" Well, keep in mind that we are all born with what I call being "orally fixated." It is a survival mechanism for us as infants to want to put something in our mouth. So when someone is smoking, part of what is the addicting behavior—not the addicting chemicals, but the addicting behavior—is the hand to mouth. This would be a great place to put in air-popped popcorn. Three cups of air-popped popcorn is only 100 calories, and she would be able to do the hand to mouth. The other thing is I would recommend chewing gum because the minute that you are going to try and eat something, you have to take gum out of your mouth to do that, so it becomes a point of behavioral modification. I think that might be some tips for her. It is a struggle for someone coming off of a nicotine addiction to not gain weight, so again, this is one of those strategies where you've got to plan your foods.

In beverages, what are the long-term impacts of diet soda and its associated chemicals on our health? Keep in mind that this category of nonnutritive sweeteners, things like aspartame and sucralose, marketing under Equal and Splenda, these chemicals must be tested before they went into the food supply. So for example, we talked about this GRAS list, generally regarded as safe. So sucrose and fructose are on the GRAS list, where NutraSweet and Splenda had to be tested before they went on the market. So the challenge is, may you have an individual adverse reaction to one of those nonnutritive sweeteners? The answer is sure. Again, we're all individuals, but in terms of long-term safety, keep in mind that moderation rules.

Our bodies love to drive down the middle of the road and they really don't like to be in the ditch. So if you said to me, "I really would love to have a diet soda in the middle of the afternoon, but I only drink one per day" your body is so unbelievably resilient that the science is going to support having an adverse reaction from that is not going to be a problem. But the science would not support if you decided in your wisdom that you were going to drink 10 diet sodas a day. Again, dose matters, so moderation is key. The unfortunate thing is that in our society, moderation doesn't sell. If we talk about moderate success, we're all looking for exceptional success, so I think that term "moderate" doesn't resonate well with the American consumer.

What about vitamin waters? Are they making them better for you? Are they great for you? I've got a couple of things with vitamin waters. First and foremost, rarely do Americans have real overt vitamin deficiencies. I'm not saying it doesn't occur because it certainly can, but it's not common for an average healthy, well person, eating a really great diet, to have a really significant deficiency in a vitamin. The challenge is, because these vitamin waters or any of the enhanced waters that are flavored, the majority of them are going to be flavored with some form of sugar. So the challenge is now what you're doing in an effort to get a vitamin supplement, you're adding more sugar. Now, certainly, there are ones out there that are lower in calories, so I think the challenge becomes, is this something that you really want to do? But I will tell you, I really wish that I would have made that up because it's been such a popular trend. It has been a real seller with Americans. The disconnect here is not all of us have a vitamin deficiency.

Another frequently asked question, is there such a thing as too little stomach acid? The answer is absolutely yes. There is a condition that's known as "achlorhydria," where you don't make enough stomach acid. We think of stomach acid as a bad thing, and it's not. Stomach acid kills bacteria, it activates thiamin, and it activates iron, and so too little stomach acid is not such a great thing. So I think the challenge is when we hear words like "acid" or we hear things that kind of get our attention, we always assume physiologically that they're bad, and in this case, we need to have some stomach acid.

"My parents have lost their sense of taste as they've aged. Is there anything that we can do to improve their eating?" Make sure that the food is flavorful. Again, depending on their overall state of health, you may need to add back some salt to their diet in order to get them to enjoy their food.

We've come to the end of this course. I want to share some final tips with you, or reminders on what it's going to take to help you to make good nutrition decisions every day. First and foremost, I'm going to tell you to eat for balance and color. All the nutrition that we need, for the majority of Americans, comes from the way that we organize our plate. Half of our plate should be fruits and vegetables, one-quarter should be lean protein, and one-quarter should be whole grain. Somehow along the way, we've wanted to make it more than that, but eating for balance and color is so important, as well as the colors of the rainbow on your plate. Colors don't mean pink bubblegum, ice cream, and golden French fries. What we're really talking about are the colors of the rainbow that come from fruits and vegetables and grain.

Another key takeaway point is that calorie control, not the newest diet on the market, is a lifelong solution. This requires you to identify where you are the weakest and create a strength. And so that's the ultimate goal in terms of overall lifetime weight management.

Also, I will always tell you to watch out for the shine. If a food is shiny on salads or pasta or meat, all sorts of dishes, they've generally added oil, and this means extra fats and oils that most of us don't need at all. So again, an ordering tip for you when you go out to dinner is ask for things to be grilled dry, sauces on the side, and you can save a significant amount of calories and still enjoy dining out with family and friends.

Remember to read labels with portion size in mind, speaking of which, watch your portion size. Eat like a child. I've mentioned before that children are blessed with eating when they're hungry and stopping when they're full. So the key strategy is maybe you fill your plate and you challenge yourself to leave a little bit left. Get used to throwing away those last couple of bites of food. Stop when you could have a few more bites, but stop before you get to that Thanksgiving fullness.

Move. Exercise is important for any good nutritional plan. We are supposed to, as human beings, move. Our bodies crave movement like they crave good nutrition. Remember, we're supposed to enjoy our foods. It's not about a nutrient. It's not about an ingredient. My ultimate definition of good nutrition is essential nutrients in the right amount plus, and underscore the "plus" here, it's the foods you love because you are you. Don't make a plan to give up something that you absolutely enjoy. Think about how you can integrate it in moderate amounts.

I will tell you, it has been a pleasure to serve as your guide through this journey to wellness. I hope with the information we've shared during this course you will be better equipped to make the best possible diet and nutrition choices for yourself and your family for a long and healthy life. Thank you very much.

Glossary

ABC model of behavior: A model to help you to manage the events that trigger behaviors and the factors that reinforce them. A is the antecedent, the event, that might trigger B, the behavior, which is followed by C, the consequences.

acanthosis nigricans: A skin disease that can be an indication of insulin resistance. Characterized by hyperpigmentation where the skin bends, such as at the knuckles, neck, breast tissue, and fat folds.

active enzyme: Enzymes that help you use your metabolic pathways a little more effectively by accelerating chemical reactions.

adequate intake (AI): For items for which there is no recommended daily allowance established, the National Academy of Sciences sets an adequate intake.

albumin: A protein that transports drugs, vitamins, and minerals.

alpha-tocopherol: The most common form of vitamin E in food (as d-isomer) and in supplements (as dl-isomer).

amino acids: The 20 building blocks of protein. They assemble the necessary proteins following instructions from our genes.

amylase: An enzyme that digests carbohydrate.

anabolic hormone: A hormone that helps to build.

angina: Severe chest pain generally considered to be from a lack of blood supply or oxygen to the heart muscle; it can be stable or unstable.

anthropometrics: Measuring the body.

atherosclerosis: Damage to the walls of the arteries.

Atkins diet: A low-carbohydrate, ketogenic diet that allows you to eat whatever you want as long as it is from protein-containing foods.

basal metabolic rate (BMR): The amount of calories that you need at rest for those functions that are not under your voluntary control. Responsible for approximately 60%–75% of the calories you need per day.

beta cell: The type of cell that makes insulin in the pancreas; a direct consumer of vitamin D.

beta-glucan: The thicker fibers that are found in oatmeal; they lower your cholesterol and support the immune function.

bile: A fluid made by the liver and stored in the gall bladder; it is needed for the emulsification of fat.

bile stasis: Occurs when bile is stored in the gallbladder for too long and there is rapid development of gallstones.

bioavailability: The amount of a nutrient that your body can absorb and utilize.

biomarker: A distinctive biological substance or indicator found in body fluids or tissues and used as a sign of a normal or abnormal process or condition.

Bitot's spots: Superficial white or gray patches occurring on the eye membrane due to deficiency of vitamin A.

blood pressure: The force of the blood pumping against the arterial walls. Normal blood pressure is 120/80 millimeters of mercury. The top number is systolic pressure, which is the force of the blood when the heart beats; the bottom number is diastolic pressure, which represents the force in between heart beats.

BOD POD: A machine that uses air displacement to assess how much of your weight is lean mass versus body fat. Body fat percentage should be less than 30% for women and less than 20% for men.

body mass index (BMI): The gold standard of population-based measurements of overweight; there is a useful BMI calculator at http://www.cdc.gov. Take your weight in pounds, multiply it by 703, and divide by your height in inches squared; a BMI of less than 24.9 is considered normal weight, between 25 and 29.9 is overweight, and greater than 30 is obese.

calorie: A unit of measure that estimates how much energy is metabolized.

carbohydrate: A nutritional powerhouse that fuels the central nervous system and exercising muscle; it is composed of carbon, hydrogen, and oxygen.

central obesity: An accumulation of excess fat around the abdomen.

cerebrovascular accident: Often known as a stroke; an interruption in the blood supply to the brain in which brain tissue is damaged and there is a subsequent loss of brain function. Symptoms include dizziness, severe headaches, nausea, and vomiting. There are 2 kinds of strokes: thrombotic and hemorrhagic.

cholesterol: A fat-soluble alcohol that can be consumed but is predominantly made in the liver.

coenzymes: Small molecules that combine with larger compounds to form active enzymes.

combining proteins: A method to balance out the essential amino acids missing in incomplete proteins.

complete proteins: Proteins that contain all of the essential amino acids that we need to build new proteins. They are usually found in animal products such as milk, cheese, chicken, fish, and red meat, but also found in soybean.

complex carbohydrates: Groups of carbohydrates known as polysaccharides; they take longer to be broken down into their component parts than simple carbohydrates do and therefore are a healthier choice.

congestive heart failure: A form of cardiovascular disease in which structural or functional problems impair the heart's ability to provide adequate blood flow to the rest of the body.

coronary artery disease: A condition in which plaque in the blood vessels builds up and restricts blood flow, which deprives the heart muscle of oxygen.

C-reactive protein: A measure of inflammatory response; the higher your C-reactive protein, the greater your inflammatory response. A more sensitive measure is the high sensitivity C-reactive protein (hs-CRP).

diabetes: *See* **type 1 diabetes, type 2 diabetes**.

diet: What you eat. You can modify your diet to meet a particular interest or health goal, but the word "diet" does not imply weight reduction.

Dietary Approaches to Stop Hypertension (DASH) diet: A diet that focuses on a high content of fruits, vegetables, and low-fat dairy products as well as a low fat composition. It can lower blood pressure in some people to the same extent as drug therapy.

dietary fiber: Nondigestible carbohydrate; it comes from the lignins: the woody portions of plants.

dietary (daily) reference intakes (DRI): Recommended intakes for individuals developed by the Institute of Medicine's Food and Nutrition Board.

dry beriberi: A disease marked by nervous system damage, with no fluid accumulation, due to thiamin deficiency.

edema: Swelling due to fluid retention.

endogenous cholesterol synthesis: The cholesterol produced in your liver, which is almost always enough to meet the body's needs.

enzyme: A protein that facilitates something to happen. In the case of salivary amylase, it facilitates the breaking down of carbohydrate.

enzyme cofactor: A chemical-reducing agent or antioxidant in both intracellular and extracellular reactions.

ergogenic: Increasing capacity for activity.

essential amino acids: Amino acids that you must have in your diet because your body cannot produce them. They include histidine, leucine, isoleucine, lysine, methionine, phenylalanine, threonine, tryptophan, and valine.

fats: Also known as lipids; the most energy dense of all the macronutrients, at 9 calories a gram. They are made up of carbon, hydrogen, and oxygen and function as an energy source, thermal insulator, hunger depressor, and vitamin carrier.

fat-soluble vitamins: Vitamins that are absorbed and stored in the body's fat stores or adipose tissue; these include vitamins A, D, E, and K. Toxic reactions can occur at much lower multiples of the recommended dietary allowances than with water-soluble vitamins.

ferritin: An iron-containing protein in cells that is a measure of your stored iron; sources include the oils of coldwater fish and flaxseed oil.

functional fiber: Nondigestible carbohydrate; the gummy fiber found in foods like oatmeal.

functional food: The American Dietetic Association defines a functional food as one that moves beyond necessity to provide additional health benefits that may reduce disease risk or promote optimal health.

g: Gram.

generally regarded as safe (GRAS): A designation given by the Food and Drug Administration to food additives generally recognized by experts to be safe.

ghrelin: A hormone that stimulates appetite.

glycemic index: A measurement of how quickly blood sugar rises after the ingestion of a particular carbohydrate food.

gynecomastia: Swelling of breast tissue in men.

Hamwi equation: Used to calculate ideal body weight. For women, allocate 100 lb for the first 5 ft of height, and allocate 5 lb for each inch over 5 ft For men, allocate 106 lb for the first 5 ft, and allocate 6 lb for each inch over 5 ft.

heart attack: An acute episode of heart disease due to decreased blood supply to the heart muscle.

hematopoiesis: Formation of blood components.

heme iron: Dietary iron that is found mainly in iron products.

hemoglobin: The protein on red blood cells that is responsible for oxygen transport; its partner, myoglobin, is the protein found in muscle tissue.

hemorrhagic stroke: A stroke defined as bleeding into the brain.

heterocyclic amines: The charred byproducts of grilling.

high-density lipoprotein (HDL) cholesterol: A blood protein that removes surplus cholesterol and fat from tissues, including the arterial wall; the higher your HDL, the lower your heart disease risk. There is an inverse relationship between triglycerides and HDL.

homocysteine: A highly reactive sulfur-containing amino acid that may increase in the blood as a result of heightened consumption of protein-rich foods and insufficient consumption of vitamin-rich foods. May contribute to damage to the lining of the arterial wall, which can lead to fatal blockages.

hydrochloric acid: A digestive acid in your stomach that denatures proteins.

hydrogenation: The process manufacturers of trans fat use to make the fat more solid; they add hydrogen to the double bonds in unsaturated fat. The consequence of hydrogenation is that they are twisting the molecule.

hypercalcemia: Elevated blood calcium.

hyperkalemia: A potassium excess most often caused by abnormal kidney or renal functioning, resulting in ineffective elimination from the body.

hypertension (or **high blood pressure)**: A blood pressure consistently higher than 140/90 millimeters of mercury. It can lead to congestive heart failure, heart attack, stroke, arterial aneurism, and chronic renal failure.

hypoalbuminemic malnutrition: Low albumin in the blood that can be caused by a stress response to a physical insult.

hyponatremia: An electrolyte abnormality due to low sodium levels from overhydration. It can cause the brain to swell and is characterized by lethargy and confusion, muscle twitching, and seizures; coma and death can occur.

ideal body weight: Calculated using the Hamwi equation (*See also* **Hamwi equation**).

incomplete protein: Proteins that are missing an essential amino acid or adequate amounts of amino acids. They are usually found in bread, nuts, rice, beans, and vegetables.

indoles: Found in cruciferous vegetables, they downregulate the production of one of the stages of cell division in the cancer process and act as negative estrogen regulators.

Glossary

296

insulin: An anabolic hormone responsible for getting glucose and other essential nutrients into cells.

integrative medicine: Medicine that treats the whole person and his or her lifestyle and encompasses the physical, psychological, and spiritual self.

international units (IU): A unit of measurement. When tested according to an internationally accepted biological procedure, it is the quantity of a hormone, toxin, or vitamin that creates a specific effect.

intrinsic factor: A compound secreted by parietal cells in the stomach that absorbs vitamin B_{12} from food, which helps prevent pernicious anemia.

inulin: A significant prebiotic that is a fiber compound; its by-products are fructo-oligosaccharides (FOS) and galacto-oligosaccharides (GOS).

keratinization: Thickening of cells.

ketogenic: Causing your body to burn fat faster than you can get rid of the waste products.

lactase: An enzyme on the tips of villi that digests lactose (milk sugar), so it can be absorbed.

leptin: A hormone that signals that the body has had enough food.

limiting amino acid: A missing essential amino acid that stops protein synthesis.

lipoprotein: The compound formed when lipids are bound to a carrier protein to allow the transport of the lipid through blood; cholesterol is at the core of these lipoprotein structures.

low-calorie diets: Diets under 1000 calories a day of mostly high-quality, protein-containing foods, such as Medifast; individuals that have severe clinical obesity may be candidates.

low-carbohydrate diet: Advocates of this diet suggest restricting carbohydrate to 20 g or fewer a day.

low-density lipoprotein (LDL) cholesterol: A blood protein that carries fat for deposition in cells, including the smooth muscle cells of your arterial walls; increased LDL levels are associated with a higher risk of heart disease.

macular degeneration: An eye disease involving the gradual loss of vision that develops especially in the elderly.

mcg: Microgram.

mean corpuscular volume (MCV): The size of the red blood cell; if you have small red blood cells, chances are you have an iron deficiency; if your red blood cells are large, you might have a deficiency of B_{12} or folic acid.

medical food: As defined by the Orphan Drug Act, "A food which is formulated to be consumed or administered enterally under the supervision of a physician and which is intended for the specific dietary management of a disease or condition for which distinctive nutritional requirements, based on recognized scientific principles, are established by medical evaluation."

metabolic syndrome: A clustering of risk factors including an increase in blood sugar and triglycerides, a decrease in HDL, an increase in blood pressure, and the accumulation of body fat. This is our early warning system that type 2 diabetes is on the way.

metabolite: A substance produced or used during metabolism.

metabolomics: A comprehensive profiling of individual metabolites including food metabolites or metabolites in your body processes.

mg: Milligram.

mono- and disaccharides: Simple sugars that contain either 1 or 2 sugars.

monounsaturated fats: Compounds that have only one double bond in a molecule; they are liquid at room temperature but get thick or viscous in the refrigerator. These can be considered heart-healthy.

mucin layer: The layer than lines the stomach and protects it by preventing it from digesting itself.

myelin sheath: The protective membrane in the central nervous system.

neurotransmitters: Chemicals that carry signals between nerve cells.

nonessential amino acids: Under circumstances of wellness, you can make nonessential amino acids in your body; they include alanine, arginine, asparagine, aspartic acid, cysteine, glutamine, glutamic acid, glycine, proline, serine, and tyrosine.

nonheme iron: Dietary iron that is found in grains and plants.

obesity: Any body mass index of greater than 30. The 3 different types of obesity that have been defined are hypercellular, hypertrophic, and hyperplastic.

omega-3 fatty acids: Highly unsaturated fat needed for the production of hormone-like compounds known as prostaglandins. Must be consumed in the diet.

omega-6 fatty acids: These tend to be overconsumed in the American diet and can increase inflammation. They are found in meat, corn oil, safflower oil, and sunflower oil.

organic: Something that has carbon as part of its structure.

organic food: A legally defined term that describes the way farmers cultivate and process agricultural products.

osteopenia: A bone mineral density value score of -1.0 to -2.5.

osteoporosis: A disorder characterized by weak and porous bones and a bone mineral density score of less than −2.5.

overfat: A condition in which body mass index may be normal, but more weight is body fat.

overload principle: That in order to get stronger, you have to make the muscle do more work than it can; overloading the muscle allows it to adapt.

overweight: A BMI of between 25 and 29.9.

oxygen radical absorbance capability (ORAC): A ranking system that gives a number to a food based on its ability to scavenge free radicals.

pancreatic lipase: An enzyme that digests fat.

Peyer's patches: Immune-secreting lymphoid tissues that are within the deepest recesses of the villi.

polyphenols: A group of compounds that may inhibit LDL oxidation, which stops arterial plaque formation. They are found in red wine, grape juice, dark berries, and cherries.

polyunsaturated fats: Compounds that have 2 or more double bonds in a molecule; they are liquid at room temperature.

prebiotics: Nondigestible food components that support the growth or activity of probiotics.

prehypertension: A blood pressure from 121/81 to 139/89 millimeters of mercury.

probiotic: Healthy bacteria added to foods; they can be found in yogurt.

prostaglandins: Hormone-like compounds formed from omega-3 fatty acids; they act as anti-inflammatories.

protein: From the Greek word *proteios*, meaning "primary." Protein can be found in every tissue in the body; its main function is to build and repair tissue.

psyllium fiber: The fiber that is found in many high-fiber breakfast cereals and in Metamucil; many commercial products designed for the treatment of constipation are based on psyllium.

recommended daily allowance (RDA): The dietary intake level you should have every day. It is sufficient to meet the requirements of nearly 98% of healthy individuals in particular life stages and gender groups.

rhodopsin: A pigment in the eyes' rods that is necessary to see black and white at night; vitamin A is a necessary constituent.

sarcopenia: The loss of about 3% of muscle mass per decade associated with aging; it contributes to a poor quality of life and increases the tendency to add body fat.

saturated fats: Long carbon fatty-acid chains that have no double bond because the whole molecule is saturated with hydrogen ions. Saturated fats are white and solid in their visible form.

standard of identity: A U.S. government regulation that sets the standards for foods to be labeled in a specific way.

stanol esters: Plant stanols that act as cholesterol mimics and attach to the cholesterol receptor in your gut to prevent the absorption of cholesterol.

statin resins: Medications that lower cholesterol by preventing it from being made in the liver; many studies suggest that statin resins can reduce the risk of a first heart attack.

steatorrhea: The malabsorption of fat that sometimes occurs as a result of genetic disorders, which can also result in severe vitamin states.

sweat rate: The number of pounds lost in physical activity. Each pound lost is 16 ounces of sweat; to rehydrate, you need about 16 to 24 ounces of fluid.

thermic effect of food: The calories it takes to digest your food.

thrombotic stroke: Occurs when an embolism breaks off and causes a blockage somewhere in the brain, most often due to the formation of a blood clot within a vessel.

total cholesterol: Composed of subfractions of other types of cholesterol; it is used as a screening tool.

total energy expenditure: How many calories you burn; determined by your basal metabolic rate, the thermic effect of food, and your physical activity level.

total energy intake: The number of calories you take in, composed of protein, fat, and carbohydrate.

total fiber: Defined by the Food and Nutrition Board of the Institute of Medicine as both dietary fiber and functional fiber.

trans fats: Unsaturated vegetable oils that manufacturers try to make more solid so they last longer.

transaminase: An enzyme that helps in the synthesis of nonessential amino acids.

triglycerides: Dietary fats that are made up of 3 fatty acids esterified to a glycerol backbone. More than 90% of the fat in our body is in this form, as is most of the fat in food.

type 1 diabetes: An autoimmune disorder in which the individual does not produce any insulin because the beta cells are no longer functioning; the individual is obligated to take insulin for the rest of his or her life.

type 2 diabetes: The most common form of diabetes, in which the body makes insulin, but it is not being effectively used by the body. Diagnosed in those with a fasting blood sugar greater than 126 milligrams per deciliter or an oral glucose tolerance test greater than 200.

underwater weighing: Also known as hydrostatic weighing; a method of measuring body composition.

unsaturated fats: Fats in which there are double bonds between the carbon molecules; they exist as monounsaturated and polyunsaturated fats.

vegan: A diet where all animal-based foods are eliminated.

villi: Small, finger-like projections that increase the surface area of the small intestine. On the tips of the villi are enzymes that digest sugar; within the recesses of the villi are Peyer's patches.

vitamins: Organic substances that must be consumed in the diet or through supplementation (the exception is vitamin D). Thirteen different vitamins have been classified into 2 major categories: fat soluble and water soluble; vitamins may be natural or synthetic.

voluntary movement: Movements such as fidgeting that are not exercise; also known as nonexercise activity thermogenesis (NEAT).

water-soluble vitamins: Vitamins that are dispersed in general in body fluids, not stored to any great extent, and probably need to be consumed on a daily basis. These include vitamin C and the B vitamins; if the diet contains less than 50% of the recommended value for a water-soluble vitamin, deficiencies can begin to appear within approximately 4 weeks.

wet beriberi: A disease marked by cardiac damage and fluid retention due to thiamin deficiency.

Bibliography

Afman, L., and M. Muller. "Nutrigenomics: From Molecular Nutrition to Prevention of Disease." *Journal of the American Dietetic Association* 106 (2006): 569–576.

Ahn, J., U. Peters, D. Albanes, et al. "Serum Vitamin D Concentration and Prostate Cancer Risk: A Nested Case-Control Study." *Journal of the National Cancer Institute* 100 (2008): 796–804.

Aiyer, H. S., M. V. Vadhanam, R. Stoyanova, et al. "Dietary Berries and Ellagic Acid Prevent Oxidative DNA and Modulate Expression of DNA Repair Genes." *International Journal of Molecular Sciences* 9 (2008): 327–341.

Ajani, U., C. H. Hennekens, A. Spelsburg, and J. E. Manson. "Alcohol Consumption and Risk of Type 2 Diabetes Mellitus among U.S. Male Physicians." *Archives of Internal Medicine* 160 (2000): 1025–1030.

American Academy of Family Physicians website. http://www.aafp.org.

American Cancer Society. "Can Cancer Be Prevented?" http://www.cancer.org/docroot/CRI/content/CRI_2_4_2x_Can_cancer_be_prevented.asp?sitearea=.

American College of Sports Medicine. "Guidelines for Healthy Adults under Age 65." http://www.acsm.org/AM/Template.cfm?Section=Home_Page&TEMPLATE=/CM/HTMLDisplay.cfm&CONTENTID=7764 (accessed April 15, 2009).

American Dietetic Association. "Nutrition and You: Trends 2008." http://www.eatright.org/ada/files/Overall_Findings_ADA_Trends_2008.pdf.

———. "Position of the American Dietetic Association: Fat Replacers." *Journal of the American Dietetic Association* 105 (2005): 266–275.

————. "Position of the American Dietetic Association: Use of Nutritive and Nonnutritive Sweeteners." *Journal of the American Dietetic Association* 104 (2004): 255–275.

————. "Ten Ways to Cut Calories." http://www.eatright.org/cps/rde/xchg/ada/hs.xsl/home_9698_ENU_HTML.htm.

American Dietetic Association website. http://www.eatright.org.

American Heart Association. "Diet and Lifestyle Recommendations." http://www.americanheart.org/presenter.jhtml?identifier=851.

————. "Risk Factors You Can't Change." http://www.americanheart.org/presenter.jhtml?identifier=3054454#heredity.

American Heart Association website. http://www.americanheart.org.

American Society of Interventional and Therapeutic Neuroradiology. "Brain Aneurysm Symptoms/Diagnosis." http://www.brainaneurysm.com/aneurysm-symptoms.html.

Arsianoglu, S., G. E. Mroro, J. Schmitt, et al. "Early Dietary Intervention with a Mixture of Prebiotic Oligosaccharides Reduces the Incidence of Allergic Manifestations and Infections during the First Two Years of Life." *Journal of Nutrition* 138 (2008): 1091–1095.

Auborn, K. J., S. Fan, and L. Goodwin. "Indole-3-Carbinol as a Negative Regulator of Estrogen." *The Journal of Nutrition* 133 (2003; suppl. 7): 2470S–2475S.

Bae, J.-M., A. J. Lee, and G. Guyatt. "Citrus Fruit Intake and Stomach Cancer Risk: A Quantitative Systematic Review. *Gastric Cancer* 11 (2008): 23–32.

Benbrook, C., X. Zhao, J. Yanez, et al. "New Evidence Confirms the Nutritional Superiority of Plant-Based Organic Foods." http://www.organiccenter.org/reportfiles/5367_Nutrient_Content_SSR_FINAL_V2.pdf (accessed April 8, 2009).

Bisset, N. G., and M. W. Wichtl, eds. *Herbal Drugs and Phytopharmaceutcials.* Stuttgart, Germany: MedPharm GmbH Scientific Publishers, 1994.

Bjelakovic, G., D. Nikolava, R. G. Simonetti, and C. Gluud. "Antioxidant Supplements for the Prevention of Gastrointestinal Cancers: A Systematic Review and Meta-Analysis." *Lancet* 364 (2004): 1219–1228.

Bloomgarden, Z. T. "Type 2 Diabetes in the Young: The Evolving Epidemic." *Diabetes Care* 27 (2004): 998–1004.

Blumenthal, M., ed. *The Complete German Commission E Monographs Therapeutic Guide to Herbal Medicine.* Austin, TX: American Botanical Council, 1998.

Bodybuilding.com website. http://www.bodybuilding.com.

Bolland, M. A., P. A. Barber, and R. N. Doughty. "Vascular Events in Healthy Older Women Receiving Calcium Supplementation." *British Medical Journal* 336 (2008): 226–227.

Bolton, M., A. Van der Straten, and C. R. Cohen. "Probiotics: Potential to Prevent HIV and Sexually Transmitted Infections in Women." *Sexually Transmitted Diseases* 35 (2008): 214–225.

Bouchard, N. C., M. A. Howland, H. A. Grellar, et al. "Ischemic Stroke Associated with Use of Ephedra Free Dietary Supplement Containing Synephrine." *Mayo Clinic Proceedings* 80 (2005): 541–545.

Bright, G. "Low-Calorie Sweeteners—From Molecules to Mass Markets." In *Low Calorie Sweeteners: Present and Future*, edited by A. Corti, 3–8. Basel, Switzerland: S. Karger AG, 1999.

Broeder, C. E., et al. "The Effects of Either High-Intensity Resistance or Endurance Training on Resting Metabolic Rate." *The American Journal of Clinical Nutrition* 55 (1992): 802–810.

Brown, A. *Understanding Food: Principles and Preparation.* 2nd ed. Belmont, CA: Wadsworth/Thompson Learning, 2004.

Brown, J. *Nutrition Now.* 4th ed. Belmont, CA: Thomson Wadsworth, 2005.

Burke, Cindy. *To Buy or Not to Buy Organic: What You Need to Know to Choose the Healthiest, Safest, Most Earth-Friendly Food.* New York: Marlowe, 2007.

Centers for Disease Control and Prevention. "Diabetes Data and Trends." http://www.cdc.gov/diabetes/statistics/prev/national/figpersons.htm.

———. "FastStats: Heart Disease." http://www.cdc.gov/nchs/fastats/heart.htm.

Charlton, O., and M. K. Sawyer-Morse. "Effect of Fat Replacement on Sensory Attributes of Chocolate Chip Cookies." *Journal of the American Dietetic Association* 96, no. 12 (1996): 1288–1290.

Clarke, K., et al. "Promotion of Physical Activity in Low-Income Mothers Using Pedometers." *Journal of the American Dietetic Association* 107 (2007): 962–967.

ConsumerLab.com. "Product Review: Probiotic Supplements." http://www.consumerlab.com/reviews/Probiotic_Supplements_Including_Lactobacillus_acidophilus_Bifidobacterium_and_Others/probiotics/ (accessed April 30, 2009).

Cook, N. R., E. Obarzanek, and J. A. Cutler. "Joint Effects of Sodium and Potassium Intake on Subsequent Cardiovascular Disease." *Archives of Internal Medicine* 169 (2009): 8–15.

Dansinger, M. L., J. A. Gleason, J. L. Griffith, et al. "Comparison of the Atkins, Ornish, Weight Watchers and Zone Diets for Weight Loss and Heart Disease Risk Reduction: A Randomized Trial." *JAMA* 293 (2005): 43–53.

DeBusk, R. "Diet-Related Disease, Nutritional Genomics, and Food and Nutrition Professionals." *Journal of the American Dietetic Association* 109, no. 3 (2009): 410–413.

DeBusk, R., C. Fogarty, J. Ordovas, and K. Kornman. "Nutritional Genomics in Practice: Where Do We Begin?" *Journal of the American Dietetic Association* 105 (2005): 589–598.

Driskell, J. A., M. C. Schake, and H. A. Detter. "Using Nutrition Labeling as a Potential Tool for Changing Eating Habits of University Dining Hall Patrons." *Journal of the American Dietetic Association* 108, no. 12 (2008): 2071–2076.

Duyff, Roberta Larson. *American Dietetic Association Complete Food and Nutrition Guide*. Hoboken, NJ: Wiley, 2006.

Dziezak, J. D. "Fats, Oils, and Fat Substitutes." *Food Technology* 43, no. 7 (1989): 66–74.

Elliott, S. S., N. L. Keim, J. S. Stern, K. Teff, and P. J. Havel. "Fructose, Weight Gain, and the Insulin Resistance Syndrome." *American Journal of Clinical Nutrition* 76 (2002): 911–922.

Ellis, K. A., G. Innocent, D. Grove-White, et al. "Comparing the Fatty Acid Composition of Organic and Conventional Milk." *Journal of Dairy Science* 89 (2006): 1938–1950.

Elmer, G. W., C. M. Surawicz, and L. V. McFarland. "Biotherapeutic Agents. A Neglected Modality for the Treatment and Prevention of Selected Intestinal and Vaginal Infections." *JAMA* 275 (1996): 870–876.

Environmental Protection Agency. "Consumer Factsheet on: Nitrates/Nitrites." http://www.epa.gov/safewater.dwh/c-ioc/nitrates.html (accessed April 8, 2009).

Environmental Working Group. "Grow Wiser about Buying Organic Foods." http://www.ewg.org (accessed April 8, 2009).

Eskin, Michael, and Snait Tamir. *Dictionary of Nutraceuticals and Functional Foods*. Boca Raton, FL: CRC Press, 2005.

Espy, M. "Ensuring a Safer and Sounder Food Supply." *Food Technology* 48, no. 9 (1994): 91–93.

Ferguson, L. "Nutrigenomics Approaches to Functional Foods." *Journal of the American Dietetic Association* 109 (2009): 425–458.

Finkelstein, E. A., I. C. Fiebelkorn, and G. Wang. "National Medical Spending Attributable to Overweight and Obesity: How Much, and Who's Paying?" *Health Affairs* W3 (2003): 219–226.

Florez, J. C. "Clinical Review: The Genetics of Type 2 Diabetes: A Realistic Appraisal in 2008." *Journal of Clinical Endocrinology & Metabolism* 93 (2008): 4633–4642.

Food and Nutrition Board, Institute of Medicine. *Dietary Reference Intakes: Applications in Dietary Assessment*. Washington, DC: National Academies Press, 2000.

———. *Dietary Reference Intakes for Energy, Carbohydrate, Fiber, Fat, Fatty Acids, Cholesterol, Protein and Amino Acids*. Washington, DC: National Academies Press, 2002.

———. *Dietary Reference Intakes for Vitamin A, Vitamin K, Arsenic, Boron, Chromium, Copper, Iodine, Iron, Manganese, Molybdenum, Nickel, Silicon, Vanadium, and Zinc*. Washington, DC: National Academies Press, 2000.

———. *Dietary Reference Intakes for Water, Potassium, Sodium, Chloride, and Sulfate*. Washington, DC: National Academies Press, 2005.

Food and Nutrition Board, and National Research Council. *Recommended Dietary Allowances*. 10th ed. Washington, DC: National Academies Press, 1989.

Food Marketing Institute. "FMI Backgrounder: Natural and Organic Foods." http://www.fmi.org/media/bg/natural_organic_foods.pdf (accessed April 8, 2009).

Ford, E. S., W. H. Giles, and W. Dietz. "Prevalence of the Metabolic Syndrome among U.S. Adults: Findings from the Third National Health and Nutrition Examination Survey." *JAMA* 287 (2002): 356–359.

Foster-Powell, K., S. H. A. Holt, and J. C. Brand-Miller. "International Table of Glycemic Index and Glycemic Load Values." *American Journal of Clinical Nutrition* 76 (2002): 5–56.

Gallus, S., et al. "Artificial Sweeteners and Cancer Risk in a Network of Case-Control Studies. *Annals of Oncology* 18 (2007): 40–44.

Garrow, J. S., A. Ralph, and William Philip Trehearne James. *Human Nutrition and Dietetics.* 10th ed. Edinburgh, Scotland: Churchill Livingstone, 2000.

Genser, D. "Food and Drug Interaction: Consequences for the Nutrition/ Health Status." *Annals of Nutrition and Metabolism* 52 (2008; suppl. 1): 29–32.

German, J. B., S. Watkins, and L. B. Fay. "Metabolomics in Practice: Emerging Knowledge to Guide Future Dietetic Advice toward Individualized Health." *Journal of the American Dietetic Association* 105 (2005): 1425–1432.

Giacco, R., G. Clemente, D. Luongo, et al. "Effects of Short-Chain Fructo-Oligosaccharides on Glucose and Lipid Metabolism in Mild Hypercholesterolaemic Individuals." *Clinical Nutrition* 23 (2004): 331–340.

Gilroy, C. M., J. F. Steiner, and T. Byers. "Echinacea and Truth in Labeling." *Archives of Internal Medicine* 163 (2003): 699–704.

Gonzalez-Periz, A., R. Horrillo, N. Ferre, et al. "Obesity-Induced Insulin Resistance and Hepatic Steatosis Are Alleviated by Omega 3 Fatty Acids:

A Role for Resolvins and Protectins." *FASEB Journal* 23, no. 6 (2009): 1946–1957.

Groff, J., and S. Gropper. *Advanced Nutrition in Human Metabolism.* 3rd ed. Belmont, CA: Wadsworth/Thompson Learning, 2000.

Gross, L. S., L. Li, E. S. Ford, and S. Liu. "Increased Consumption of Refined Carbohydrates and the Epidemic of Type 2 Diabetes." *American Journal of Clinical Nutrition* 79 (2004): 774–779.

Guthrie, J., and J. Morton. "Food Sources of Added Sweeteners in the Diets of Americans." *Journal of the American Dietetic Association* 100 (2000): 43–51.

Harrison C. "The (Still) High Cost of Organic Foods." http://www.alternet.org/environment/24821?page=1 (accessed April 8, 2009).

Harvard School of Public Health website. http://www.hsph.harvard.edu.

Hasler, C. M., A. C. Brown, and American Dietetic Association. "Position of the American Dietetic Association: Functional Foods." *Journal of the American Dietetic Association* 109 (2009): 735–746.

Heaney R. P., K. Raffety, M. S. Dowell, and J. Bierman. "Calcium Fortification Systems Differ in Bioavailability." *Journal of the American Dietetic Association* 105, no. 5 (2005): 807–809.

Heasman, Michael, and Julian Mellentin. *The Functional Foods Revolution: Healthy People, Healthy Profits?* Sterling, VA: Earthscan, 2001.

Heller, Lorraine. "Mintel Identifies Major Trends to Impact Food Industry." Foodproductiondaily.com, May 9, 2006. http://www.foodproductiondaily.com/Supply-Chain/Mintel-identifies-major-trends-to-impact-food-industry.

Hrovat K. B., et al. "The New Food Label, Type of Fat, and Consumer Choice. A Pilot Study." *Archives of Family Medicine* 3, no. 8 (1994): 690–695.

Hu, F., M. J. Stampfer, and J. E. Manson. "Trends in the Incidence of Coronary Artery Disease and Changes in Diet and Lifestyle in Women." *The New England Journal of Medicine* 343 (2000): 530–537.

Huffnagle, Gary B., and Sarah Wernick. *The Probiotics Revolution: The Definitive Guide to Safe, Natural Health Solutions Using Probiotic and Prebiotic Foods and Supplements.* New York: Bantam Dell, 2008.

"Hypertension: What Works? Drugs Do—But a New Diet Is Sometimes Enough." *Consumer Reports*, May 1999.

Insel, Paul M., R. Elaine Turner, and Don Ross. *Discovering Nutrition.* 3rd ed. Sudbury, MA: Jones & Bartlett, 2009.

International Food Information Council. "Consumer Attitudes Toward Functional Foods/Foods For Health—Executive Summary. http://ific.org/research/funcfoodsres07.cfm (accessed April 7, 2009).

———. "Functional Foods: Attitudinal Research. http://www.ific.org/research/funcfoodsres02.cfm (accessed April 7, 2009).

———. "Qualified Health Claims Consumer Research Project Executive Summary." http://www.ific.org/research/qualhealthclaimsres.cfm (accessed April 7, 2009).

———. "Tailoring Your Diet to Fit Your Genes: A Global Quest." http://www.ific.org/foodinsight/2006/jf/genesfi106.cfm (accessed April 7, 2009).

Jentjens, R. L., and A. E. Jeukendrup. "Effects of Pre-Exercise Ingestion of Trehalose, Glactose and Glucose on Subsequent Metabolism and Cycling Performance." *European Journal of Applied Physiology* 88 (2003): 459–465.

Jin, L., M. Qi, and A. Anderson. "Indole-3-Carbinol Prevents Cervical Cancer in Human Papilloma Type 16 Transgenic Mice." *Cancer Research* 59 (1999): 3991–3997.

Kajiyama, Y., K. Fuji, H. Takeuchi, et al. "Gingko Seed Poisoning." *Pediatrics* 109 (2002): 325–327.

Kaput, J. "Diet-Disease Gene Interactions." *Nutrition* 20, no. 1 (2004): 26–31.

Kaput, J., and R. L. Rodriguez. "Nutritional Genomics: The Next Frontier in the Postgenomic Era." *Physiological Genomics* 16 (2004): 166–177.

Kavanaugh, C. J., P. R. Trumbo, and K. C. Ellwood. "The U.S. Food and Drug Administration's Evidence-Based Review for Qualified Health Claims: Tomatoes, Lycopene, and Cancer." *Journal of the National Cancer Institute* 99 (2007): 1074–1085.

Kawamori, T., et al. "Chemopreventive Effect of Curcumin, a Naturally Occurring Anti-Inflammatory Agent, During the Promotion/Progression Stages of Colon Cancer." *Cancer Research* 59 (1999): 597–601.

Klis, J. B. "Continuing Trend: Reducing Fat and Calories." *Food Technology* 47, no. 1 (1993): 152.

Knowler, W. C., E. Barrett-Conner, S. E. Fowler, et al. "Reduction in the Incidence of Type 2 Diabetes with Lifestyle Intervention or Metformin." *The New England Journal of Medicine* 346 (2002): 393–403.

Kristal, A. R., et al. "Predictors of Self-Initiated, Healthful Dietary Change." *Journal of the American Dietetic Association* 101, no. 9 (2001): 997.

Kummeling I., C. Thijs, M. Huber, et al. "Consumption of Organic Food and the Risk of Atopic Disease during the First 2 Years of Life in the Netherlands." *British Journal of Nutrition* 99, no. 3 (2008): 598–605.

Langemead, L., R. M. Feakins, S. Goldthorpe, et al. "Randomized, Double Blind, Placebo Controlled Trial of Oral Aloe Vera Gel for Ulcerative Colitis." *Alimentary Pharmacology & Therapeutics* 19 (2004): 739–747.

Lara-Villoslada, F., M. Olivares, and S. Sierra. "Beneficial Effects of the Probiotic Bacteria Isolated from Breast Milk." *British Journal of Nutrition* 98 (2007; suppl. 1): S96–S100.

Lee, D. H., A. R. Folsom, and D. R. Jacobs. "Dietary Iron Intake and Type 2 Diabetes Incidence in Postmenopausal Women: The Iowa Women's Health Study." *Diabetologia* 47 (2004): 185–194.

Lee, I. M. "Physical Activity and Cancer Prevention—Data from Epidemiologic Studies. *Medicine and Science in Sports and Exercise* 35 (2003): 1823–1872.

Levine, J. A., N. L. Eberhardt, and M. D. Jensen. "Role of Nonexercise Activity Thermogenesis in Resistance to Fat Gain in Human." *Science* 283 (1999): 212–214.

Liong, M. T. "Safety of Probiotics: Translocation and Infection." *Nutrition Review* 66 (2008): 192–202.

Mahan, K., and S. Stump. *Krause's Food, Nutrition, and Diet Therapy.* 11th ed. Philadelphia: Elsevier, 2004.

Mayo Clinic Staff. "Organic Foods: Are They Safer? More Nutritious?" http://www.mayoclinic.com/health/organic-food (accessed April 8, 2009).

Mayo Clinic website. http://www.mayoclinic.com.

McArdle, William D., Frank I. Katch, and Victor L. Katch. *Exercise Physiology: Energy, Nutrition, and Human Performance.* 6th ed. Baltimore, MD: Lippincott Williams and Wilkins, 2007.

McFarland, L. V., and S. Dublin. "Meta-Analysis of Probiotics for the Treatment of Irritable Bowel Syndrome." *World Journal of Gastroentergology* 14 (2008): 2650–2661.

McNutt, K. "Common Sense Advice to Food Safety Educators." *Nutrition Today* 32, no. 3 (1997): 128–133.

Mead, Paul S., et al. "Synopses: Food Related Illness and Death in the United States." *Emerging Infectious Diseases* 5, no. 5 (1999): 607–625.

Mela, D. J. "Nutritional Implications of Fat Substitutes." *Journal of the American Dietetic Association* 92, no. 4 (1992): 472–476.

Michos, E. D., and R. S. Blumenthal. "Prevalence of Low Low-Density Lipoprotein Cholesterol with Elevated High Sensitivity C-Reactive Protein in the U.S.: Implications of the Jupiter Study." *Journal of the American College of Cardiology* 553 (2009): 931–935.

"Mineral Deficiency and Toxicity." *Merck Manual of Patient Symptoms.* http://www.merck.com/mmpe/sec01/ch005/ch005a.html (accessed October 2, 2009).

Mital, B. K., and S. K. Garg. "Anticarcinogenic, Hypocholesterolemin, and Antagonistic Activities of *Lactobacillus acidophilus. Critical Reviews in Microbiology* 21 (1995): 175–214.

Mitchell, A. E., Y.-J. Hong, E. Koh, et al. "Ten-Year Comparison of the Influence of Organic and Conventional Crop Management on the Content of Flavonoids in Tomatoes." *Journal of Agricultural and Food Chemistry* 55 (2007): 6154–6159.

Moriarty, Naithani R., and B. Surve. "Organosulfur Compounds in Cancer Chemoprevention." *Mini Reviews in Medicinal Chemistry* 7 (2007): 827–838.

Moshfegh, Alanna J., James E. Friday, Joseph P. Goldman, and Jaspreet K. Chug Ahuja. "Presence of Inulin and Oligofructose in the Diets of Americans." *The Journal of Nutrition.* http://jn.nutrition.org/cgi/content/full/129/7/1407S (accessed May 1, 2009).

Mukherjee, A., D. Speh, E. Dyck, and F. Diez-Gonzalez. "Preharvest Evaluation of Coliforms, *Escheria coli, Salmonella,* and *E. coli* O157:H7 in Organic and Conventional Produce Grown by Minnesota Farmers." *Journal of Food Protection* 67 (2004): 894–900.

Mullins, R. J., and R. Heddle. "Adverse Reactions Associated with Echinacea: The Australian Experience." *Annals of Allergy, Asthma & Immunology* 88 (2002): 42–51.

Myers, J., A. Kaykha, S. George, et al. "Fitness versus Physical Activity Patterns in Predicting Mortality in Men." *The American Journal of Medicine* 117 (2004): 912–918.

National Advisory Committee on Microbiological Criteria for Foods. "Hazard Analysis and Critical Control Point Principles and Application Guidelines: Adopted August 14, 1997." http://www.cfsan.fda.gov/~comm/nacmcfp.html#princ.

National Institutes of Health. "National Digestive Diseases Information Clearinghouse." http://digestive.niddk.nih.gov/statistics/statistics.htm (accessed October 2, 2009).

Nayga, R. M., Jr. "Retail Health Marketing: Evaluating Consumers' Choice for Healthier Foods." *Health Marketing Quarterly* 16, no. 4 (1999): 53–65.

Neuhouser, M. L., A. R. Kristal, and R. E. Patterson. "Use of Food Nutrition Labels Is Associated with Lower Fat Intake." *Journal of the American Dietetic Association* 99, no. 1 (1999): 45–53.

Northwestern University. "Nutrition Fact Sheets." http://www.feinberg.northwestern.edu/nutrition/fact-sheets.html (accessed October 1, 2009).

Nowack, R. "Cranberry Juice—A Well Characterized Folk-Remedy against Bacterial Urinary Tract Infection." *Wien Med Wochenschr* 157 (2007): 325–330.

NuVal. "How It Works. FAQs: The NuVal System." http://www.nuval.com/pages/Faq.aspx.

Organic Monitor. "The Global Market for Organic Food and Drink." http://www.organicmonitor.com/700140.htm (accessed April 8, 2009).

Palomer, X., J. M. Gonzalez-Clemente, F. Blanco-Vaca, and D. Mauricio. "Role of Vitamin D in the Pathogenesis of Type 2 Diabetes Mellitus." *Diabetes Obesity and Metabolism* 10 (2008): 185–197.

Peters, U., M. F. Leitzmann, N. Chatterjee, et al. "Serum Lycopene, Other Carotenoids, and Prostate Cancer Risk: A Nested Case-Control Study in the Prostate, Lung, Colorectal, and Ovarian Cancer Screening Trial." *Cancer Epidemiology, Biomarkers & Prevention* 16, no. 5 (2007): 962–968.

Pillai, U., J. Muzaffar, and S. Sen. "Grapefruit Juice and Verapamil: A Toxic Cocktail." *Southern Medical Journal* 102 (2009): 308–309.

Pittler, M. H., M. Kieser, and U. Holscher. "Ginkgo Biloba Extract for the Treatment of Intermittent Claudication: A Meta Analysis of Randomized Trials. *The American Journal of Medicine* 108 (1998): 276–281.

Pszczola, D. E. "Functional Ingredients Enhance Value of Low-Fat Foods and Micro Waved Foods." *Food Technology* 46, no. 4 (1992): 116.

Quigley, E. M. "Bacteria: A New Player in Gastrointestinal Motility Disorders-Infections, Bacterial Overgrowth, and Probiotics." *Gastroenterology Clinics of North America* 6 (2007): 735–748.

Raben, A., T. Vasilaras, C. Moller, and A. Astruup. "Sucrose Compared with Artificial Sweeteners: Different Effects on Ad Libitum Food Intake and Body Weight after 10 Wk of Supplementation in Overweight Subjects." *American Journal of Clinical Nutrition* 76 (2002): 721–729.

Reilly, P., and R. DeBusk. "Ethical and Legal Issues in Nutritional Genomics." *Journal of the American Dietetic Association* 108 (2008): 36–40.

Rembialkowska, E. "Review: Quality of Plant Products from Organic Agriculture." *Journal of the Science of Food and Agriculture* 87 (2007): 2757–2762.

Reynolds, P., S. E. Hurley, R. B. Gunier, et al. "Residential Proximity to Agricultural Pesticide Use and Incidence of Breast Cancer in California, 1988–1997." *Environmental Health Perspectives* 113 (2005): 993–1000.

Riley, Dan. "Texans' Rep Rules." http://www.houstontexans.com/mobile/story.asp?story_id=3680 (accessed September 30, 2009).

Rodriguez, N. R., N. M. DiMarco, S. Langley, American Dietetic Association, Dietitians of Canada, and American College of Sports Medicine. "Position of the American Dietetic Association, Dietitians of Canada, and the American College of Sports Medicine: Nutrition and Athletic Performance." *Journal of the American Dietetic Association* 109 (2009): 509–527.

Rossi, F., I. Bertuzzi, S. Comizzoli, et al. "Preliminary Survey on Composition and Quality of Conventional and Organic Wheat." *Italian Journal of Food Science* 4 (2006): 355–366.

"Selenium." Vitamin & Herb University website. http://www.vitaminherbuniversity.com/topic.asp?categoryid=2&topicid=1028.

Shalev, E., S. Battino, E. Weiner, et al. "Ingestion of Yogurt Containing *Lactobacillus acidophilus* Compared with Pasteurized Yogurt as Prophylaxis for Recurrent Candidal Vaginitis and Bacterial Vaginosis." *Archives of Family Medicine* 5 (1996): 593–596.

Shearer, M. J. "Role of Vitamin K and Gla Proteins in the Pathophysiology of Osteoporosis and Vascular Calcification." *Current Opinion in Clinical Nutrition and Metabolic Care* 3 (2000): 433–438.

Shelton, R. C., M. B. Keller, A. Gelenburg, et al. "Effectiveness of St. John's Wort for Major Depression: Randomized Controlled Trial." *JAMA* 285 (2001): 1978–1986.

Shurbsole, M. J., F. Jin, Q. Dai, et al. "Dietary Folate Intake and Breast Cancer Risk: Results from the Shanghai Breast Cancer Study." *Cancer Research* 61 (2001): 7136–7141.

Silverthorn, Dee Unglaub. *Human Physiology, An Integrated Approach.* 4th ed. Menlo Park, CA: Benjamin/Cummings, 2007.

Smart Choices Program website. http://www.smartchoicesprogram.com/ index.html.

Stalenhof, A. F., and J. de Graf. "Association of Fasting and Nonfasting Serum Triglycerides with Cardiovascular Disease and the Role of Remnant-Like Lipoproteins and Small Dense LDL." *Current Opinion in Lipidology* 19, no. 4 (2008): 355–361.

Stevinson, C., M. H. Pittler, and E. Ernst. "Garlic for Treating Hypercholesterolemia: A Meta Analysis of Randomized Controlled Trials." *Annals of Internal Medicine* 133 (2000): 420–429.

Sturm, R. "Increases in Morbid Obesity in the U.S.A.: 2000–2005." *Public Health* 121 (2007): 492–496.

Tahiri, M., J. C. Tressol, J. Arnaud, et al. "Five-Week Intake of Short-Chain Fructo-Oligosaccharides Increases Intestinal Absorption and Status of Magnesium in Postmenopausal Women." *The Journal of Bone and Mineral Research* 16 (2001): 2152–2160.

Thomas, D., and E. J. Elliott. "Low Glycaemic Index, or Low Glycaemic Load Diets for Diabetes Mellitus." *Cochrane Database of Systematic Reviews.* January 21, 2009 (1): CD006296.

Tindale, H. A., R. B. Davis, R. S. Phillips, and D. M. Eisenberg. "Trends in Use of Complementary and Alternative Medicine by U.S. Adults 1997–2002." *Alternative Therapies in Health and Medicine* 11 (2005): 42–49.

Tornwall, M. E., J. Virtamo, P. A. Korhonen, M. J. Virtanen, P. R. Taylor, D. Albanes, and J. K. Huttunen. "Effect of Alpha-Tocopherol and Beta-Carotene Supplementation on Coronary Heart Disease during the 6-Year Post-Trial Follow-Up in the ATBC Study." *European Heart Journal* 25 (2004): 1171–1178.

Trujillo, E., C. Davis, and J. Milner. "Nutrigenomics, Proteomics, Metabolomics, and the Practice of Dietetics." *Journal of the American Dietetic Association* 106 (2006): 403–413.

U.S. Cancer Statistics Working Group. "United States Cancer Statistics: 1999–2005 Incidence and Mortality Web-Based Report." http://www.cdc.gov/uscs.

U.S. Department of Health and Human Services, and U.S. Department of Agriculture. *Dietary Guidelines for Americans, 2005.* http://www.health.gov/DietaryGuidelines/dga2005/document/default.htm (accessed October 2, 2009).

U.S. Food and Drug Administration. "Consumer Nutrition and Health Information." http://www.cfsan.fda.gov/~dms/fdnewlab.html.

———. "FDA 101: Health Fraud Awareness." http://www.fda.gov/ForConsumers/ProtectYourself/HealthFraud/default.htm (accessed October 5, 2009).

———. "Food Labeling and Nutrition: Dietary Supplements Label Claims." http://www.cfsan.fda.gov/~dms/labstruc.html (accessed April 7, 2009).

———. "Food Labeling and Nutrition: Food Labeling and Nutrition Overview." http://www.cfsan.fda.gov/~dms/qatrans2.html#s3q3.

———. *Guidance for Industry: A Food Labeling Guide.* http://www.fda.gov/Food/GuidanceComplianceRegulatoryInformation/GuidanceDocuments/FoodLabelingNutrition/FoodLabelingGuide/default.htm (accessed October 1, 2009).

———. "How to Understand and Use the Nutrition Facts Label." http://www.cfsan.fda.gov/~dms/foodlab.html.

———. "Legislation." http://www.fda.gov/opacom/laws/DSHEA.html.

————. "Orphan Drug Act." http://www.fda.gov/RegulatoryInformation/ Legislation/FederalFoodDrugandCosmeticActFDCAct/Significant AmendmentstotheFDCAct/OrphanDrugAct/default.htm (accessed September 30, 2009).

USDA Agricultural Research Service. "USDA National Nutrient Database for Standard Reference, Release 21." http://www.ars.usda.gov/Services/ docs.htm?docid=17477 (accessed October 1, 2009).

USDA Economic Research Service. "U.S. Food Consumption Up 16 Percent Since 1970." http://www.ers.usda.gov/AmberWaves/November05/ Findings/USFoodConsumption.htm.

USDA Food Safety and Inspection Service. "Safe Food Handling: A Consumer's Guide to Food Safety; Severe Storms and Hurricanes (2008)." http://www.fsis.usda.gov/Fact_Sheets.

Van Helden, Y. G., J. Keijer, A. M. Knaapen, S. G. Heil, J. J. Briedé, F. J. van Schooten, and R. W. Godschalk. "Beta-Carotene Metabolites Enhance Inflammation-Induced Oxidative DNA Damage in Lung Epithelial Cells." *Free Radical Biology & Medicine* 46, no. 2 (2009): 299–304.

Versteegen, M., and S. Neubauer. "Organic Foods: Are They a Safer, Healthier Alternative?" *Nutrition in Complementary Care* 11 (2008): 1–31.

Villegas, R., Y. T. Gao, Q. Dai, et al. "Dietary Calcium and Magnesium Intakes and the Risk of Type 2 Diabetes: The Shanghai Women's Health Study." *The American Journal of Clinical Nutrition* 89 (2009): 1059–1067.

Vogler, B. K., and E. Ernst. "Aloe Vera: A Systematic Review of Its Clinical Effectiveness." *The British Journal of General Practice* 49 (1999): 823–828.

Wadden, T. A., D. S. West, R. H. Neiberg, et al. "One Year Weight Loss in the Look Ahead Study: Factors Associated with Success." *Obesity* 17 (2009): 713–722.

Watson, J. L., R. Hill, P. W. Lee, et al. "Curcumin Induces Apoptosis in HCT-116 Human Colon Cancer Cells in a p21-Independent Manner." *Experimental and Molecular Pathology* 84, no. 3 (2008): 230–233.

Weihrauch, M. R., and V. Diehl. "Artificial Sweeteners—Do They Bear a Carcinogenic Risk? *Annals of Oncology* 15 (2004): 1460–1465.

Welsh, J. A., M. E. Cogswell, S. Rogers, H. Rockett, Z. Mei, and L. M. Grummer-Strawn. "Overweight Among Low-Income Preschool Children Associated with the Consumption of Sweet Drinks: Missouri, 1999–2002." *Pediatrics* 115 (2005): 223–229.

Whelton, S. P., A. Chin, Xue Xin, and He Jiang. "Effect of Aerobic Exercise on Blood Pressure: A Meta-Analysis of Randomized, Controlled Trials." *Annals of Internal Medicine* 136 (2002): 493–503.

Wickline, N. M. "Prevention and Treatment of Acute Radiation Dermatitis: A Literature Review." *Oncology Nursing Forum* 31 (2004): 237–247.

Williams, C. M., and K. G. Jackson. "Inulin and Oligofructose: Effects on Lipid Metabolism from Human Studies." *British Journal of Nutrition* 87 (2002; suppl. 2): S261–S264.

Williams, P. "Consumer Understanding and Use of Health Claims for Foods." *Nutrition Review* 63, no. 7 (2005): 256–264.

Wilsgaard, T., H. Shcrimer, and E. Arnesen. "Impact of Body Weight on Blood Pressure with a Focus on Sex Differences: Tromos Study, 1986–1995." *Archives of Internal Medicine* 160 (2000): 2847–2853.

Wolf, I., J. J. van Croonenborg, H. C. Kemper, et al. "The Effect of Exercise Training Programs on Bone Mass: A Meta Analysis of Published Controlled Trials in Pre- and Postmenopausal Women." *Osteoporosis International* 9 (1999): 1–12.

World Health Organization. "Obesity and Overweight." http://www.who.int/dietphysicalactivity/publications/facts/obesity/en (accessed April 14, 2009).

Yamaguchi, P. "Japan's Nutraceuticals Today—Functional Foods Japan 2006." http://www.npicenter.com/anm/templates/newsATemp.aspx?articleid=15160 &zoneid=45 (accessed April 5, 2009).

Credible Nutrition Websites

General Information:

American College of Sports Medicine: http://www.acsm.org.
American Dietetic Association: http://www.eatright.org.
Centers for Disease Control and Prevention: http://www.cdc.gov.
Food and Nutrition Information Center of the U.S. Department of Agriculture: http://fnic.nal.usda.gov.
Food Safety and Inspection Service of the U.S. Department of Agriculture: http://www.fsis.usda.gov.
Mayo Clinic: http://www.mayoclinic.com.
National Institutes of Health: http://www.nih.gov.
U.S. Food and Drug Administration: http://www.fda.gov.

More Specific Topics and Lecture-Related Topics:

Lecture 1

Portion Distortion Quiz:
Part 1: http://hp2010.nhlbihin.net/oei_ss/PD1/slide1.htm.
Part 2: http://hp2010.nhlbihin.net/oei_ss/PDII/slide1.htm.

Fast Food Nutrition Facts:
http://www.dietfacts.com/fastfood.asp.

Nutrition for Kids:
http://www.eatright.org/ada/files/Snacks_for_Kids_English.pdf.
http://www.eatright.org/ada/files/Wendys.pdf.

Lecture 2

Health Fraud of the Past and Present and Tips for Recognizing Health Fraud: http://www.fda.gov/fdac/features/2006/606_fraud.html.

Lecture 4

Body Mass Index and Daily Caloric Needs Calculator:
http://www.nutritiondata.com/tools/calories-burned.

Lecture 5

Hydration Needs and Tips—Staying Hydrated and Rehydrating:
http://www.mckinley.uiuc.edu/Handouts/hydrate_needs_exercise.html

Lecture 6

Carbohydrates, Lipids, and Protein Explained:
http://www.mckinley.uiuc.edu/handouts/macronutrients.htm.

Glycemic Index and Carbohydrate Needs Explained:
http://www.hsph.harvard.edu/nutritionsource/what-should-you-eat/
carbohydrates-full-story/index.html.

Lecture 7

Importance of Fiber and Your Daily Fiber Needs:
http://www.hsph.harvard.edu/nutritionsource/what-should-you-eat/
fiber-full-story/index.html.

Lecture 8

Carbohydrates, Lipids, and Protein Explained:
http://www.mckinley.uiuc.edu/handouts/macronutrients.htm.

Protein Intake for Athletes:
http://www.vanderbilt.edu/ans/psychology/health_psychology/Protein.htm.

Lecture 9

Dietary Fats Explained:
http://www.eatright.org/ada/files/Martek_Fact_Sheet.pdf.
http://www.eatright.org/ada/files/DIETARY_FATS.pdf.
http://www.americanheart.org/presenter.jhtml?identifier=3045789.
http://www.americanheart.org/presenter.jhtml?identifier=3049042.

Lecture 10

Vitamins—Functions in the Body and Food Sources:
http://www.nwhealth.edu/healthyU/eatWell/vitamins_2.html.

Lecture 14

Directory of Common Foods and Nutrients Contained: http://www.ars.usda.gov/Services/docs.htm?docid=17477.

Lecture 15

Minerals—Sodium and Potassium:
http://www.health.gov/DietaryGuidelines/dga2005/document/html/chapter8.htm.
http://www.eatright.org/ada/files/Mrs_Dash.pdf.

Lecture 17

Nutrition and Cardiovascular Disease:
http://www.eatright.org/ada/files/Metamucil_Fact_Sheet.pdf.
http://www.americanheart.org/presenter.jhtml?identifier=3038016.

Lecture 19

General Information:
http://www.nhlbi.nih.gov/health/public/heart/hbp/dash/new_dash.pdf.
http://www.eatright.org/cps/rde/xchg/ada/hs.xsl/media_3053_ENU_HTML.htm.

Lecture 20

Overweight, Overfat, and Obesity:
http://www.eatright.org/ada/files/Popular_Diets_Reviewed_2007.pdf.
http://www.americanheart.org/presenter.jhtml?identifier=4639.

Lecture 21

Personalized eating plans and interactive tools to help plan and assess your food choices:
http://www.mypyramid.gov/.

Credible Nutrition Websites

Lecture 22

General Information:
http://www.americanheart.org/presenter.jhtml?identifier=3044757.
http://www.americanheart.org/presenter.jhtml?identifier=3044762.
http://www.hsph.harvard.edu/nutritionsource/more/type-2-diabetes/.
http://www.diabetes.org/about-diabetes.jsp.

Lecture 23

National Weight Control Registry: http://www.nwcr.ws.
American Dietetic Association: http://www.eatright.org.

Lecture 24

MD Anderson Cancer Center: http://www.mdanderson.org.
Memorial Sloan-Kettering Cancer Center: http://www.mskcc.org.

Alcohol Intake and Breast Cancer:
http://www.breastcancer.org/tips/nutrition/ask_expert/2005_01/question_07.jsp.

Nutrition and Cancer Prevention:
http://www.eatright.org/ada/files/Eat_Your_Way_to_Better_Health.pdf.
http://prevention.cancer.gov/prevention-detection/lifestyle.

Lecture 25

General Information:
http://www.eatright.org/ada/files/Purdue_Fact_Sheet.pdf.

Lecture 27

Food Safety and Inspection Service of the U.S. Department of Agriculture:
http://www.fsis.usda.gov/factsheets/.
Food Safety and Food-Borne Illnesses:
http://www.foodsafety.gov/.

Lecture 28

Understanding and Reading Food Labels:
http://www.mayoclinic.com/health/nutrition-facts/NU00293.
http://www.eatright.org/ada/files/Shop_Smart.pdf.

Lecture 29

General Information:
http://www.eatright.org/cps/rde/xchg/ada/hs.xsl/advocacy_934_ENU_
HTML.htm.

Information on Specific Foods:
http://www.eatright.org/ada/files/Almond_Fact_Sheet.pdf.
http://www.eatright.org/ada/files/Barley.pdf.
http://www.eatright.org/ada/files/Hershey_Fact_Sheet.pdf.
http://www.eatright.org/ada/files/Mango.pdf.
http://www.eatright.org/ada/files/The_Plant_Sterol_Story.pdf.

Lecture 30

General Information:
http://www.eatright.org/ada/files/Supplements.pdf.
http://www.eatright.org/cps/rde/xchg/ada/hs.xsl/advocacy_3311_ENU_
HTML.htm.
http://www.umm.edu/altmed/.

Lecture 31

General Information:
http://www.ams.usda.gov/AMSv1.0/nop.

Lecture 33

Healthy Eating on the Run:

http://www.eatright.org/ada/files/Healthy_Eating_on_the_Run.pdf.

Rate Your Plate, by the University of Connecticut's Team Nutrition: http://www.sp.uconn.edu/~cthompso/.

Log your food intake and exercise: http://www.fitday.com/.

Determine the calories in the food you eat: http://www.calorieking.com/.

DETERMINE questionnaire for older people from the American Academy of Family Physicians: http://www.aafp.org/afp/980301ap/edits.html.

Lecture 34

American College of Sports Medicine: http://www.acsm.org.

Body Mass Index and Daily Caloric Needs Calculator (Estimate): http://www.nutritiondata.com/tools/calories-burned.

Sports Nutrition and Nutrition for the Physically Active Adult: http://www.gssiweb.com.

Lecture 36

American Dietetic Association: http://www.eatright.org.
American College of Sports Medicine: http://www.acsm.org.

Notes